Conversations with the Soul

First published by Muswell Hill Press, London, 2018

This edition by Aeon Books, London, 2023

© 2018. Andrew Powell

Andrew Powell has asserted his right under the Copyright, Design and Patents Act 1988 to be identified as the author of this work. All rights reserved. No part of this publication may be reproduced without prior permission of Aeon Books Ltd.

British Library CIP Data available

ISBN: 978-1-913274-49-8

Conversations with the Soul

A Psychiatrist Reflects:
Essays on Life, Death and Beyond

Dr Andrew Powell

AEON

For my beloved family:
my wife Melinda,
my children Anna, Joshua, Hugo and Flora,
and grandchildren Charlotte, Tom, Oscar, Lilla, Jake and Emilia

Contents

Acknowledgements — ix
Foreword — xi
Preface — xv

1. The Contribution of Spirit Release
   Therapy to Mental Health — 1
2. Why Must We Suffer? A Psychiatrist Reflects — 13
3. Spirituality and Psychiatry – Crossing the Divide — 25
4. Whither the Soul of Psychiatry? — 39
5. Past Life Memory – A Key to Understanding the Self? — 57
6. Soul-Centred Psychotherapy — 73
7. Healing and the Wounded Psyche — 89
8. Open Heart, Open Mind: Conversing with the Soul — 101
9. Recovery and Well-Being: The Search for the Soul — 111
10. Vocation Under Duress — 125
11. The Whole Patient — 141
12. What Does It Mean to be Human? — 151
13. The Place of Medicine in Today's World — 155
14. Technology and Soul in the 21st Century — 161
15. Modernity and the Beleaguered Soul — 181
16. Helping Patients Tell Their Story: Narratives of
    Body, Mind and Soul — 193
17. Prejudice – Can We Live Without It? — 211

Index — 221

Acknowledgements

I wish to express my thanks again to Dr Tim Read for the publication of this second volume of my papers by Muswell Hill Press and to Kasia Trojanowska for her editorial assistance. My thanks also for permissions given by the publishers of papers that had earlier found their way into print. In the exacting task of revising the papers for this book, I am especially grateful to my wife Melinda, both for her discerning eye and for constant support.

I earlier recorded in *The Ways of the Soul* my appreciation of the many people who have helped me to find an understanding of life in general and my own in particular. I remain indebted to all who have accompanied me this far – patients, colleagues and friends, and my beloved family. I must own that life has its rough edges too, and not all encounters in life are congenial, yet I have found on occasions that opposition has taught me what I most needed to learn!

Turning from the personal to the transpersonal, our human lives mirror the succession of the seasons and this stage of my passing years could fairly be described as autumn. During the summer of my life, it came forcibly to me how we are all playing our part in an interweaving of events that unfold to reveal life's greater design, which moved me to a profound and lasting sense of gratitude. I am reminded of the acclaimed quote from Meister Eckhart: 'If the only prayer we ever say in our lives is "Thank You", that will be enough!'

Gratitude must have its recipient, and it is instructive to ask 'Who am I thanking?' I have found that the question is not for the mind but for the heart. Desirous for the best of both worlds, I give thanks for the fellowship of souls as we journey together through the year, and to my Maker, whose seasons are infinite.

Foreword

Over the past few centuries, we have reached dazzling heights of scientific, medical and technological advance, which have improved the conditions of our lives and facilitated a phenomenal expansion of our ability to express the creative genius of our species in many different fields. But we have also suffered a catastrophic loss of soul, a loss of the ancient awareness of the sacred – of the sense of participation in the life of Nature, the Cosmos, and our connection to Spirit, the spring from which all of life flows. Instead, in our secular era, the rational human mind is now given supreme value, recognising no dimension of reality beyond the physical universe, nor any form of consciousness transcendent to its own. Cut off from its roots, it has banished the unknown, unexplored, non-rational aspect of life.

There is astonishingly little awareness in our materialist culture that the psyche or soul is a vital component of consciousness and that the heart is at least as important as the brain in understanding the complex causes of mental illness. Most people have no idea that there is another aspect of themselves beyond their conscious rational mind. Science has taught them that consciousness is something produced by the physical brain and therefore does not survive the death of the physical body. The existence of the transpersonal conscious, first explored by Jung and researched since by many others in the past 70 or so years, has been largely ignored.

Consequently, our current world-view rests on the premise of our separation from, and mastery of, Nature, where the resources of the planet are unthinkingly plundered to serve the ever-growing numbers and needs of our species. In our consumerist society, people are not helped to explore the deeper meaning and purpose of life. This is why our culture is so unbalanced and why so many people, quite apart from the specific stresses of their lives, are deeply depressed and anxious. They are aware that something is amiss; something that is not being acknowledged or addressed by our culture.

A fundamental cause of mental illness is this loss of soul in our technology-addicted society and the fact that those afflicted by depression and other symptoms of distress cannot find the help they so badly need. Despite the unprecedented mass prescribing of pharmaceuticals, the epidemic of depression continues to grow apace – a sure sign that the real answer is not to be found by tampering with the chemistry of the brain.

I first met Andrew Powell in 2001 at St Thomas' Hospital in London, where we were both giving talks. I was at once struck by his calm, empathic way of addressing the audience, which immediately had everyone present listening intently. As a Jungian analyst, I was attracted to the subject matter of his talk as well as his manner of speaking. Since then, our friendship has deepened and in 2012 we organised a conference together entitled 'Seeing Beyond The Veil: The Survival of the Soul and Life Beyond Death'.

As a physician, psychiatrist and psychotherapist, Andrew has been addressing the far-reaching concerns outlined above for more than 20 years. In the preface to his first volume of papers, he writes:

> 'The medicalisation of human anguish now woven into our culture reflects a society that seems unable to stand back and ask what we are doing to ourselves, the communities in which we live and the natural world. This brings me to a further theme in these papers. What are the assumptions that we make in our post-modern world about the nature of reality? How is it that we are so conditioned by the culture of material realism that many believe that the world of the five senses is all that exists? And what does this pervasive culture of materialism do to the human spirit?'[1]

Importantly, there is now a New Story emerging in quantum physics, which tells us that the whole universe is a unified field. We live within a cosmic web of life, which underlies and connects all life forms in the universe and on our planet. Every atom of life interacts with every other atom, no matter how distant. We are connected with each other not only through the Internet but also through an immense field of consciousness, which sustains not just our world, but the entire Cosmos. As a species, we urgently need to move forward into a more advanced kind of consciousness, one that embraces this connectedness of both heart and mind.

In 1999, Andrew founded the Spirituality and Psychiatry Special Interest Group of the Royal College of Psychiatrists, which now numbers around 3000 psychiatrists. As well as engaging with the public through its website and conferences, the group has attracted the support of many mental health colleagues who had been looking for what was missing from their professional life. The success of this

---

1. Powell (2017: xvii).

group makes clear that Andrew's passionate interest in the spiritual dimension of healthcare is shared by colleagues who are frustrated by the current paradigm of mental illness.

It is immensely encouraging, as well as inspiring, to browse through the wide-ranging papers selected for this second volume. Andrew draws on a lifetime of clinical practice, as well as his personal experience of individuation or soul growth, suggesting that 'the soaring demand on mental health services calls for a soul-envisioned perspective on what humanity at its best can be, and how we might bring this about.'[2]

These papers offer us a greater understanding of why mental illness is increasing so dramatically today and why its underlying causes need to be recognised and addressed through an understanding of the soul and its needs. Andrew's work shows us how reaching out to others soul to soul is at the heart of healing the psyche, thereby enabling the human spirit to prevail.

Anne Baring
Jungian analyst
Author of The Dream of the Cosmos: A Quest for the Soul

Reference

Powell, A. (2017) *The Ways of the Soul. A Psychiatrist Reflects: Essays on Life, Death and Beyond.* Muswell Hill Press.

---

2. p. xix, this volume.

Preface

This second volume of my papers on spirituality and mental health spans the decade 2006 to 2016. Some papers were written for mental health professionals and others for a wider audience. As with the first volume, *The Ways of the Soul*, the papers are set out in chronological order and while there has been revision throughout, with additional footnotes providing updates, they are recognisably in their original form.

My premise is that spiritual awareness has far-reaching implications for the understanding and treatment of emotional disorders. Every human being must encounter suffering sooner or later. While for many this is balanced by joy in the richness and rewards of life well lived, those who come to the attention of the psychiatrist carry a burden of distress from which there can seem no escape.

Psychiatrists aim to relieve this suffering by means of two main approaches, physical therapy (most often pharmaceutical) and psychological therapy.[1] However, in no small part due to the pressure on mental health services today, the first-line treatment provided is usually pharmaceutical.

Yet human beings are infinitely more than mental mechanisms and brain neurochemistry, and the human spirit, our most precious asset, must not be left out in the cold.[2] The psychiatrist who is willing to enlist the spiritual potential of his or her patient will find a unique opportunity to explore the big questions of meaning and purpose that so often surface in the course of a breakdown. There is nothing abstruse about this, for every person has such innate wisdom ready and waiting to be used – if one only trusts in its presence and perseveres in looking for it.

My foremost concern has been to put people in touch with this wisdom, so that its influence can be brought to bear on the distress

---

1. Broadly speaking, psychological therapies work either by bringing to light unconscious mental processes (psychodynamic therapy) or by directly tackling unhelpful thought processes (cognitive–behavioural therapy).
2. In recent years, mindfulness-based cognitive therapy (MBCT) has been shown to help prevent relapse in depression. MBCT owes much to the Buddhist tradition of meditation, although in mental healthcare it is presented as a short-term therapy rather than a spiritual practice.

experienced by the mundane, everyday mind. In order for this to happen, the therapist must bear with the confusion, hurt and anger that may arise when the patient is faced with questions that may seem unanswerable, such as: 'What is my life for? What is the point of it all? Why should I (or my loved ones) have to suffer like this? How can God allow this to happen?' Throughout history, these existential questions have troubled humanity struggling to make sense of the human condition. In the case of mental disorder, such anguish painfully reveals the travails of the ego, yet it can open the way to a heartfelt conversation with the soul – an inexhaustible repository of wisdom and love.

On a different note, this volume, like the first, refers not infrequently to advances in cosmology that suggest we live in an inherently spiritual universe. Current researches into quantum field theory and holographic cosmology offer a view of the cosmos as the expression of a supreme intelligence enthusing us with life and consciousness.[3] In this case, God is going to be manifest not only in the Higgs boson but everywhere we look, not least in ourselves.[4]

Some papers included here describe how connection with soul can be made in a very personal way, while others concern the collective soul of humanity. A good deal of sorrow and misfortune is contained in the clinical examples, for such is the climate of psychiatric practice.[5] However, I trust that the narratives of hope and love that arise whenever the soul is helped to make itself known will more than compensate.

THE CONTRIBUTION OF SPIRIT RELEASE THERAPY TO MENTAL HEALTH returns to the subject of spirit attachment previously discussed in *The Ways of the Soul*. Psychiatry treats anomalous perception as nothing but a hallucination produced by the brain and little credibility is given to any other explanation. Notwithstanding, a brief account is given here of the phenomenology of spirit attachment, including demonic possession. Whatever the exact nature of the underlying process, working with compassion is essential in spirit release, whether we understand it to be a psychological therapy, a spiritual therapy, or both.

WHY MUST WE SUFFER? A PSYCHIATRIST REFLECTS starts by distinguishing between pain as a sensation and suffering that arises from

---

3. The root of enthuse is found in the Ancient Greek *én-theos* (in God).
4. The Higgs boson is an elementary particle thought to be key to the creation of mass in subatomic particles and thus to the formation of all matter. Also popularly known as the 'God particle'.
5. Names and other details cited in the case studies have been changed to protect anonymity.

the awareness of loss. Experienced first in childhood and thereafter throughout life, loss can be a spur to the maturing self but, if overwhelming, leads to withdrawal and depression. When the soul goes unheeded, loss is experienced as a dead end – for this is how the ego sees it. Yet from the soul perspective there is always a way forward, one that can bring healing and renewal of life.

SPIRITUALITY AND PSYCHIATRY – CROSSING THE DIVIDE begins with an account of my early fascination with medicine, second only to the desire to understand the workings of the mind, and thence to specialising in psychiatry and psychotherapy. I describe how my interests later led me to study healing, transpersonal psychology and soul-centred therapy, and how I set out to raise awareness of the spiritual dimension within psychiatry by means of a Spirituality and Psychiatry Special Interest Group in the Royal College of Psychiatrists.

WHITHER THE SOUL OF PSYCHIATRY? reviews the spiritual beliefs and practices of antiquity, the ecclesiastical dogma leading to the witch-hunts of the Middle Ages and, following the Age of Enlightenment, the building of asylums in the 19th century. In the 20th century, the new specialty of psychiatry, deeply preoccupied with scientific credibility, turns its back on the spiritual aspect of care – a legacy that has endured. However, a growing interest in spirituality and mental health today underlines that treating the brain is not the same as treating the person.

PAST LIFE MEMORY – A KEY TO UNDERSTANDING THE SELF? first looks at how the infant must survive and grow by means of the development of a healthy egoic self. However, in contrast to the eternal 'now' of the spiritual self, the ego is constantly occupied with its past and with threats to its future survival. In 'past life' therapy, we are shown that the afflictions of life, no matter how grievous to the ego, find understanding, healing and forgiveness in a kinder realm – one that lies beyond the compass of death.

SOUL-CENTRED PSYCHOTHERAPY illustrates by means of clinical case studies how the soul perspective can be brought to bear on the human condition. A number of different approaches are described, all of which have the same objective: helping a person to become aware of their soul presence and how to be guided by what the soul has to say. Soul consciousness brings clarity of insight unperturbed by life's upheavals, helping the patient to see their circumstances with new-found wisdom and compassion.

HEALING AND THE WOUNDED PSYCHE is a personal account of how, after some years of working in mainstream analytical psychotherapy, the writings of Carl Jung and my growing interest in a reality that transcends the limitations of physicalist science lead me to the study and practice of healing. With healing comes the deep knowledge that the unconditional love bestowed by the soul is a precious gift given to humanity to share – never more needed than now.

OPEN HEART, OPEN MIND: CONVERSING WITH THE SOUL begins by distinguishing between projection and the evolutionary importance of empathy. Empathy puts us in touch with the suffering of others and the desire to help lighten another's burden. Such is the nature of compassion. Where the ego so often divides, the soul unites; through empathy we see ourselves in the other and the other in us – the prerequisite for all soul-centred therapy.

RECOVERY AND WELL-BEING: THE SEARCH FOR THE SOUL questions the value of the diagnostic framework used in psychiatry today. Not only does a psychiatric diagnosis frequently lack both validity and reliability, but it also risks putting a label on the patient that can hinder recovery. A decisive step to recovery is in reclaiming personhood and for this, the ego needs restoring to health. The further step, which is to admit the soul, brings wholeness of self and oneness with life.

VOCATION UNDER DURESS compares conditions in the National Health Service in the 1970s with the burden of stress experienced by many healthcare staff today. Abraham Maslow's 'hierarchy of needs' is used to show how institutional malaise arises when essential preconditions are not met. In contrast, proper care of bodily needs, a sense of safety and security, experiencing kinship and working in a culture of mutual esteem and respect – all contribute to bringing about Maslow's highest level of self-actualisation, characterised by altruism, optimism and working for the common good.

THE WHOLE PATIENT explores how the wholeness of being with which we are born is inevitably challenged throughout life by adversities of one kind or another. When the threat to physical or emotional well-being is overwhelming, the ego goes into defence mode and life becomes at best something to be survived. Yet when a person is able to draw strength from the soul, adversity can be the spur to finding wholeness of self and peace of mind, so that even death can be met with gratitude for what has been and equanimity for what is to come.

WHAT DOES IT MEAN TO BE HUMAN? is a short reflection on this present moment in the time-line of the human species, when we have the means as never before to make heaven or hell on Earth. Judging by the world today, if the egoic mind is left to its own devices, humankind risks extinction. However, if the soul can take the lead, we have the chance to create a future that is worthy of the extraordinary gift of life.

THE PLACE OF MEDICINE IN TODAY'S WORLD takes a look at humankind's fervent hope that illness and disease will continue to roll back before the advance of medical science. Yet, at the same time, we adopt behaviours that bring about many of the harms we fear, whether in war or peace. No amount of medical research and technology can stop self-inflicted pain and disease – a shadow that will accompany humanity until we comprehend that all life is one, and live accordingly.

TECHNOLOGY AND SOUL IN THE 21ST CENTURY contrasts the 'top down' religious and spiritual world-views with the 'bottom up' worldview of empirical science. The fault lies not with the nature of scientific enquiry but with the abuse of derivative technologies riding on the back of profit and power. Examples of 'techno-pathology' are given that now endanger both human and planetary health and well-being. Our best hope lies in educating the ego in the ways of the soul, so becoming fully aware of the immense privilege and responsibility given to us for the future of humanity and for the whole Earth.

MODERNITY AND THE BELEAGUERED SOUL explores the social conditioning that has permeated the developed world, one in which the sacred has been largely confined to religious life, while a secular culture of material realism thrives as never before. The result has not been an abundance of human happiness. The ideology of perpetual growth founded on borrowing, consumerism and pleasure-seeking has proved to be no substitute for deeper values, meaning and purpose. The soaring demand on mental health services calls for a soul-envisioned perspective on what humanity at its best can be, and how we might bring this about.

HELPING PATIENTS TELL THEIR STORY: NARRATIVES OF BODY, MIND AND SOUL returns to the consulting room and the doctor-patient relationship. Modern medicine is indebted to the achievements of science. Nevertheless, in the case of psychiatry, person-centred care must always come first if the wounds of the psyche are to be helped to heal. Examples are given of soul narratives that arise when the patient is encouraged to bring to light the inner wisdom that is the spiritual birthright of every human being.

Prejudice – Can We Live Without It? looks at the dire impact of prejudice on the modern world. The origins of prejudice lie in the defensive mentality of the group in response to its perception of external threat, in past times no doubt serving the social evolution of our species. Now, however, the scale of global conflict and the weapons at the disposal of humankind are such that prejudice is endangering all of life as we know it. Only when humanity grasps that there is but the one life we were made to share, the essence of which is love, will prejudice be overcome.

1

The Contribution of Spirit Release Therapy to Mental Health

I will begin this discussion of a controversial treatment approach with a short case study.

> James sought help for depression and alcohol abuse. Always lacking in confidence, he had dropped out of university and found work in the art trade. When James was 28, his brother Ivor shot himself. James found the body in a nocturnal search. The family was devastated. James began to drink heavily and became chronically depressed. After many years of unsuccessful psychotherapy and medication, on the advice of a friend he requested spirit release therapy.
>
> James readily entered an altered state of consciousness and the spirit of the deceased brother, Ivor, began speaking 'through him'. Ivor explained that he wanted to move on, but that their mother's continuing need was holding him in the earth plane. Ivor was asked by the therapist to approach their mother through his guardian angel and request his release. Ivor did so, and at once found himself free to go into the Light.
>
> The contact that James made with his brother prepared him to let go of his own emotional ties with their mother. He required just two more sessions for healing. Two years later, he was happily married and working as a gardener. There has been no recurrence of depression or alcohol abuse.[1]

First published in *Light* (2006), 126(1), pp. 10–16. Reproduced with permission. Revised for conference 'Spirit Possession and Mental Health', held by BME Mental Health, London, June 2009.

---

1. Case study included by courtesy of the Spirit Release Foundation. Details of conferences, training in spirit release therapy and a list of registered practitioners are available from the Spirit Release Forum (www.spiritrelease.org).

This kind of therapeutic intervention, no matter its good outcome, is profoundly at variance with mainstream psychiatric diagnosis and treatment, and I shall be exploring some of the issues involved.

Science, Spirit and the Nature of Reality

The scientific community of today regards soul-centred therapies such as spirit release as entirely pre-rational,[2] belonging to an era of superstition overthrown by the scientific advances of the past 300 years. Furthermore, science – including mental health science – makes a clear distinction between reality and imagination. There is nothing 'out there' that is not either physical or else something imagined by the mind. Such a view holds no truck with 'attached spirits'. How could there be a spirit without a body?

This dismissal by material realism is essentially atheistic – there is no place for God[3] or angels, let alone 'earthbound spirits'. Yet the greatest scientists, such as Albert Einstein, have consistently shown awe and humility in the face of the unknown. Science may illuminate the mysterious workings of the cosmos, yet what is revealed can be compared with the pool of light shed by a street lamp at night.

Medicine, psychiatry included, works by the light of that street lamp. Illnesses of the body are diagnosed and fixed like a car that has broken down and most mental disorder, too, is treated as a disorder of brain chemistry. Advances in neuroscience, furthered by PET and fMRI brain scans, are cited in support of this approach. At the same time, science discounts subjective truth as largely irrelevant for its lack of demonstrable validity.

The neurochemical model of psychiatric disorder remains unproven to this day.[4] Nevertheless, the pharmaceutical industry capitalises heavily on the sale of medications,[5] some of them prescribed life-long.[6] Where, on the other hand, is profit to be made from purely psychological or spiritual aspects of healthcare?

Further, psychiatry is understandably reluctant to enquire into the 'paranormal'. A great deal of psychiatry has depended on agreeing what

---

2. Ellenburger (1970).
3. This was Freud's firmly held view. See Freud (1927).
4. Moncrieff (2007).
5. In 2015, global sales of antidepressants, stimulants, anxiolytics and antipsychotics were estimated at over 76 billion US dollars a year. See Dewan (2014).
6. For an in-depth review of the dangers of long-term medication, see Whitaker (2011).

is 'normal' and then evaluating in what way, and how far, the mindset of any one individual differs from the consensus view. When a person deviates sufficiently from that norm, it is called psychopathology – disease of the mind. Jesus Christ, had he lived in our time, would likely be diagnosed as suffering from delusions of grandeur. What indeed would psychiatry today make of the revelations of the saints and prophets, or of the epiphanic visions of the 14th-century acolyte, Mother Julian of Norwich?[7]

Nonetheless, instances of anomalous perception, including telepathy, precognition, deathbed visions, out-of-body and near-death experiences, continue to be reported, while past life therapy and mediumship remain subjects of intense interest to the wider public.[8] Moreover, there is now strong research evidence for psychokinesis, presentiment and distance healing, to name but a few.[9,10,11]

What kind of science would be required in order to accommodate such phenomena within its conceptual framework? Interestingly, quantum mechanics is revolutionising our concept of reality. The 'new physics' tells us there is no such thing as true objectivity, the very foundation of classical physics, indeed that there is no world of 'things' that exists independently of consciousness. There is also strong evidence that everything is connected to everything else, our universe comprising one unimaginably vast hologram.[12] More recent still, the mathematics of string theory asserts that we exist in a cosmos of at least 11 dimensions!

According to quantum mechanics, the stable and structured world of sense perception we take as consensus reality arises from what is called the 'collapse of the probability wave', generated by millions of minds over time. Yet each of us has a capacity to collapse the wave in a place of our own making, transgressing the laws of classical physics. On one notable occasion, Jesus turned water into wine![13] No matter how improbable, from the quantum perspective everything is possible.

If what we take for real is not immutable, as classical physics would have us believe, and given the evidence that consciousness is

---

7. Backhouse (1987).
8. For further discussion, see *Past Life Memory – A Key to Understanding the Self?*, this volume.
9. Schmidt (1987).
10. Radin (1997).
11. Fontana (2004).
12. For a brief update on holographic cosmology, see PhysOrg (2017).
13. John 2:1–11 *The Holy Bible*, NIV.

not only personal but also transpersonal, how may we distinguish between mental illness and communications from 'other realms', including when they might overlap? A good way to begin is to find out whether the experience being reported is enhancing or disrupting a person's life – a distinction not always easy to make, since turmoil often accompanies the process of change. Nevertheless, the aim must be to see what kind of meaning and purpose is attributed, and whether this can be beneficial.

This approach is helpful when considering mediumship. A medium should be able to choose when to be receptive to receiving communications from 'the other side of life'. The information given should be coherent and appropriate to the context, even though the phenomenology of the (hallucinated) voice or vision may be the same as for a person with a severe mental disorder. Yet the significance for health as opposed to illness is entirely different. Psychiatry does acknowledge this in ICD-10,[14] the diagnostic manual used in the UK. Under trance and possession disorders (F44.3), we find:

> '…there is a temporary loss of both the sense of personal identity and full awareness of the surroundings; in some instances the individual acts as if taken over by another personality, spirit, deity, or "force".'

Importantly, ICD-10 goes on to say that:

> 'Only trance disorders that are involuntary or unwanted, and that intrude into ordinary activities by occurring outside (or being a prolongation of) religious or other culturally accepted situations should be included here.'

Mediums can thus be reassured that the psychiatrist is not entitled to diagnose them as mentally ill. But where does this leave 'spirit attachment'? This is more difficult, since we have to bear in mind that 'attachment' is in relation to a person's vulnerability, for example, due to illness, bereavement and emotional and physical trauma, as well as constitutional sensitivity. Disorders of brain function – severe depression, drug misuse and schizophrenia – are all held to render a person susceptible, in which case an individual may be said to be both ill and suffering from intrusive spirit attachment. This is why it is essential to make a careful assessment in each case.

---

14. ICD-10, *The International Classification of Diseases*, a standardised diagnostic tool issued by the World Health Organization. See World Health Organization (1992).

The Spiritual Universe

Throughout history, all cultures that acknowledge the presence of spirit[15] have been deeply preoccupied with the relationship of the human soul to the discarnate world, not least with regard to the nature of good and evil. Is evil palpably a thing in itself and therefore to be cast out? If so, what does this suggest about the nature of the Godhead from whence it must have arisen?[16] Should we understand there to be a polarity in the human psyche, meaning that good and evil cannot exist without each other? Alternatively, is evil sheer 'ignorance', based on the failure to grasp the age-old golden rule that ultimately we are all one, and therefore that to harm another is to harm oneself?

The Abrahamic faiths have portrayed heaven as a dwelling for the virtuous, while sinners are cast into outer darkness. However, the shamanic and spiritualist traditions have always envisioned a universe of holographic correspondences, hence the ancient saying, 'as above, so below'. Emanuel Swedenborg[17] and Allan Kardec[18] most notably describe how in non-earthly realms, spirits are drawn to the plane that resonates with the level of their own spiritual development. Similarly, it is said that in life we attract spirits to us according to our 'vibration', on the same principle of sympathetic resonance that 'like attracts like'.

Great spiritual masters who embody unconditional love are attuned to the very highest vibrations. Similarly, every medium committed to working with 'light' brings through communications that are uplifting and inspiring. However, from the transpersonal perspective, human nature is such that not only the 'light' but also the shadow side of the human psyche needs to be acknowledged. When the shadow makes itself known, it is profoundly disturbing because we are being shown what we do not want to see about ourselves. Yet the shadow can be a spur to growth, for when we are confronted by it – whether from within or without – we are being given the spiritual challenge of finding light in the darkness.

---

15. I generally prefer to describe spirit as the sacred, animating principle of creation from which arises the manifest universe, and the word soul as meaning the unique expression of spirit in each individual. However, spirit release therapists generally speak of 'earthbound spirits', possibly because to use the word 'soul' suggests embodiment in physical form.
16. For a discussion of the nature of the Godhead, see *The Unquiet Self and the Search for Peace*, in Powell (2017).
17. Swedenborg (1758).
18. Kardec (1857).

Spirit Attachment

Studies of the near-death experience[19] corroborate what had previously been reported through mediumship, namely that death is a transition in which the soul leaves the physical body for worlds beyond.

However, spirit release therapists contend that a minority of those who die fail to make the transition successfully, instead becoming earthbound spirits. Such a person has died carrying fear, anger or obsessive love so strong that the spirit cannot let go of the earth plane, remaining instead in a dimension adjacent to the material world (known as the lower astral plane). For such spirits, consciousness often appears to be confined to a twilight state, with only dim awareness of the passage of time. Sometimes the spirit does not even grasp that death has occurred, particularly when violent death has left it in a state of shock.

Other spirits are unable or unwilling to let go of their earthly appetites, whether sexual or from addiction to drugs or alcohol, and will seek out and attach to someone still alive who shares their tastes. This provides the spirit with the means of satisfying its unfulfilled appetites – to the further detriment of the host, who may suffer depleted energy, loss of appetite, damage to health, relationships, career and mental disturbance to the point of suicide.[20]

It is also held that not all attaching spirits are discarnate, and that the malign influence of one living person on another should not be overlooked. Psychic attack can damage the health of the victim mentally and physically, sometimes causing severe bodily pain. The person mounting the attack may be using sorcery or witchcraft, enlisting the influence of 'demonic entities'.

This brings us back to the problem of evil. In the course of spirit release therapy, a minority of spirits, when challenged, are found never to have existed in human form. Their aim is to harass, harm and eventually destroy a person's capacity for life and love. One such archetype that frequently presents to the spirit release practitioner is that of the 'fallen angel', who, having succumbed to the power of Lucifer, abandoned the light for the dark and in doing so, lost touch with their own divinity. Such an entity can be helped to find its way back to the light.[21] However, more powerful demonic entities not only reject any therapeutic intervention, but can become extremely aggressive. Practitioners must know the limits of their competence and referral to the deliverance

---

19. See compilation by Bailey & Yates (1996).
20. Sanderson (2003).
21. An example is given in *Soul-Centred Psychotherapy*, this volume.

ministry of the Church, to an imam or a minister of another faith tradition may be appropriate.

Making an Assessment

The relationship between spiritual pathology and psychopathology can be complex; a person may present with either or both together. In my view, it is not advisable to attempt spirit release therapy where there is evident mental illness. Instability and/or fragmentation of the psyche will result at best in temporary improvement and at worst may exacerbate a complex delusional system.

When spirit release is being considered, the therapist will need to take a full history, identifying the occasion of the attachment, the nature of the vulnerability and the presenting symptoms. The language used often gives a clue, for example, the person speaking of being 'unable to move on', aware of the 'presence' of the departed loved one or of feeling 'haunted' by memories of the deceased – indeed, sometimes speaking openly of feeling 'possessed'.

In dealing with such cases, the therapist can ask the patient to look within and 'scan' for any object or presence that feels harmful or disturbing. If, for example, the patient reports finding 'black stuff in the back of my head', the therapist might say, 'You, black stuff, I want to talk with you!' This will usually provoke a response, although not always a polite one! The therapist persists with questions, such as 'How did you get in? How long have you been in there? Why are you with this person?', which elucidate the nature of the attachment and determine the course of action to be taken.[22]

Ethical good practice requires that spirit release therapy should be offered only when it is consonant with the patient's wishes. It is important to clarify with the patient what the process entails, so that informed consent can be given. This means explaining that the patient will be encouraged to sit back, letting the 'spirit' make itself known using the patient's voice and allowing the words – whatever comes – to flow spontaneously.

---

22. This method is called 'interactive', to distinguish it from the 'intuitive' approach, in which a clairvoyant practitioner will 'read' the problem, and very likely communicate with the intrusive entity by means of extra-sensory perception.

Spirit Release Therapy

The approach taken by the Spirit Release Forum is always to work compassionately with the attached spirit and to call on help from 'above' as needed. Release may be facilitated by encouraging the earthbound spirit to reflect on its former life and thereby to understand the nature of its entrapment. An empathic enquiry by the therapist generally brings about the awakening of a desire by the spirit to let go and move to the light. Sometimes the spirit becomes aware of deceased loved ones waiting for them, or angels may be summoned to take the spirit with them. As the spirit goes into the light, the patient often sighs with relief, visibly relaxing as though a palpable burden has been lifted.

When a demonic entity is encountered, many spirit release therapists take the therapeutic approach advocated by Baldwin.[23] Calling on angelic help, the entity is surrounded by a 'net of light'. Such entities show intense fear that the light will burn and so can be exhorted to retreat inwards, into their own darkness. Urged to go deeper and deeper, the entity (to its astonishment) discovers a light within, which far from burning feels wonderful! With this revelation comes a flood of remorse for the harm it has been doing. The entity can then be carried by the heavenly host into the light, where atonement can be made and forgiveness found.

An important aspect of release therapy is that once freed, the patient may need further psychological work in order to strengthen the integrity of the psyche. Entities are believed to seek a flaw in the psyche with which they can resonate – unresolved shadow complexes, or weakness of ego structure due to illness, alcohol/drugs or trauma – and a resilient, healthy psyche is the surest protection against attachment.

Spirit Release Today

How might spirit release therapy hope to be more widely acknowledged as a credible treatment approach?

There are two possibilities. The first would entail a major paradigm shift within contemporary science. Computational quantum mechanics suggests that the space-time framework of our perceptual world is nested within other dimensions and that consciousness is not epiphenomenal (created *de novo* by the brain) but primary and enduring. This would invite a reappraisal of perceptual anomalous experiences, having

---

23. Baldwin (1992).

profound cultural and religious implications for the meaning of birth, death, and existence itself. For this to happen, humanity would need to embrace a very different vision of reality – one that would doubtless be resisted in the prevailing climate of material realism.[24]

The other possibility is simply to treat spirit release as a specific psycho-spiritual intervention in those cases where such help is being sought. It has long been recognised that working with the beliefs of the patient often leads to the best result.[25] Given that the ontological status of discarnate spirits is entirely unresolved, such a pragmatic approach has certain advantages.

For clairvoyant mediums, the presence of spirits is self-evident while sceptics will claim that even the best outcome using spirit release therapy does not prove the existence of spirits. This largely fruitless argument can be avoided if the intervention is simply deemed useful for selected patients.[26] While it is desirable to know how a treatment works, it is not necessary so long as it helps the patient. Indeed, much of science is based on input and output, without knowing what really goes on in the inner workings of the black box.

Keeping an Open Mind

Newtonian physics is based on the principle of either/or (for instance, an object cannot be in two places at the same time). In the quantum domain, however, subatomic particles exist and do not exist at the same time; they can be everywhere and nowhere at once. Moreover, space, once thought to be an empty vacuum, is now known to be swarming with energies of unbelievable magnitude.[27]

Could it be that Nature in her wisdom has largely shielded us from the impact of these energies, so that our personal, everyday selves can get on with raising families, holding down jobs, living to the full emotionally and, when we have spare time, puzzling on the nature and purpose of life? Yet it seems that in an altered state of consciousness, whether through psychedelic drugs, hypnotherapy, meditation or simply stilling of the mind, we may find ourselves in touch with very different worlds.[28]

---

24. Resistance to paradigm change is an age-old feature of the human psyche. See Kuhn (2012).
25. Frank (1963).
26. The 2017 update of ICD-10 now treats 'disorders of trance and possession' as a subset of 'other dissociative and conversion disorders' (F44.89).
27. McTaggart (2001).
28. See also *Past Life Memory – A Key to Understanding the Self?*, this volume.

When someone has the misfortune to suffer from the disturbance of brain function called schizophrenia, it has been suggested that the psyche becomes porous to energies that were never intended to flood in.[29] Likewise, when the emotions of the bereaved connect them with the energies of the deceased, should we be so surprised by communications that come from 'beyond the veil'?

The eternal attribute of consciousness is a wonderful thing, but so is space-time; otherwise, our bodies would not exist and we would be deprived of the chance of growing in knowledge and wisdom through the challenges that life brings. Provided that our actions are occasioned by love, free from prejudice and tempered with humility, spirit release therapy may yet find its place as a valued contribution to mental healthcare.

References

Backhouse, H. (ed.) (1987) *Julian of Norwich: Revelations of Divine Love*. Hodder & Stoughton.
Bailey, L. & Yates, J. (1996) *The Near Death Experience*. Routledge.
Baldwin, W.J. (1992) *Spirit Releasement Therapy: A Technique Manual*. Human Potential Foundation Press.
Dewan, S.S. (2014) *Drugs for Treating Mental Disorders: Technologies and Global Markets* (BCC Market Research Report PHM074B). BCC Market Research.
Ellenburger, H. (1970) *The Discovery of the Unconscious*. Basic Books.
Fontana, D. (2004) *Is there an Afterlife?* O Books.
Franco, D.P. (1979) *Obsession* (trans. E.J. Donato & H.C. Miranda). Centro Espirita 'Caminho da Redencao'.
Frank, J. (1963) *Persuasion and Healing*. Schocken Books.
Freud, S. (1927) The future of an illusion. Reprinted [1961] in *The Standard Edition of the Complete Psychological Works of Sigmund Freud*, vol. 21 (trans. & ed. J. Strachey). Hogarth Press.
Kardec, A. (1857) *The Spirits' Book* (trans. D. Kimble). Federação Espírita Brasileira, R/J, Brazil, 2006.
Kuhn, T. (2012) *The Structure of Scientific Revolutions*. University of Chicago Press.
McTaggart, L. (2001) *The Field*. HarperCollins.
Moncrieff, J. (2007) *The Myth of the Chemical Cure: A Critique of Psychiatric Drug Treatment*. AIAA.
PhysOrg (2017) Study reveals substantial evidence of holographic universe. Available at https://phys.org/news/2017-01-reveals-substantial-evidence-holographic-universe.html (accessed 4 July 2017).
Powell, A. (2017) *The Ways of the Soul. A Psychiatrist Reflects: Essays on Life, Death and Beyond*. Muswell Hill Press.
Radin, D. (1997) *The Conscious Universe*. Harper Edge.

---

29. Franco (1979).

Sanderson, A. (2003) Spirit release therapy. What is it and what can it achieve? A clinical presentation of therapist and patient perspectives. Available at www.rcpsych.ac.uk/spsigarchive

Schmidt, H. (1987) The strange properties of psychokinesis. *Journal of Scientific Exploration*, 1, 103–118.

Swedenborg, E. (1758) *Heaven and Hell* (trans. G. Dole). Swedenborg Foundation, 2000.

Whitaker, R. (2011) *Anatomy of an Epidemic: Magic Bullets, Psychiatric Drugs, and the Astonishing Rise of Mental Illness in America.* Broadway Books.

World Health Organization (1992) *International Statistical Classification of Diseases and Related Health Problems, 10^h Revision* (ICD-10).

2

Why Must We Suffer? A Psychiatrist Reflects

Philosophers and theologians have wrestled with the problem of suffering since the dawn of civilisation, but I daresay we are no closer to finding an answer today than in the time of Lao Tsu, the Buddha, Plato, Jesus Christ or the Prophet Muhammad, for suffering and life go hand-in-hand.

Being a doctor has brought me into contact with a good deal of suffering, both physical and emotional, and so I would like to offer some reflections on the nature of suffering, the challenges it presents, and how to work with suffering in order to relieve despair and bring hope.

What is Suffering?

I will start by making the distinction between pain, which is a sensation, and suffering, which means to be aware of what pain signifies. When we lose a cherished possession, suffering arises because of the emotional significance of the loss – all the more so when living with the prospect of chronic pain or disability, or of losing what we hold dear, be it one's work or friendships. For most people, the greatest loss to be faced is the ending of life, whether one's own or that of a loved one.

Once a person has grasped that birth brings with it the inevitability of death, the desire to be well carries with it, consciously or otherwise, the fear of illness and the realisation that happiness, insofar as it depends on health, is at best ephemeral.

This poignant truth is recounted in the myth of Adam and Eve, exiled from the Garden of Eden for eating the fruit of the tree of knowledge.

Paper prepared for conference 'Suffering – What is the Point of it All?' held by the Spirituality and Psychiatry Special Interest Group at the Royal College of Psychiatrists, London, March 2007.

Their fate was to live thereafter with a yearning for the paradise they could never regain. Yet, in awakening to self-awareness and finding themselves cast out into the world of birth, sickness, ageing and death, they could begin the journey from *Homo innocens* to *Homo sapiens*.

The theme of loss informs all great art and literature. These days it also plays an important part in our understanding of mental health, and so I first want to consider how the pain of loss shapes the future of every human child.

The Trauma of Birth

To start at the beginning: before birth, we now know the baby is actively responding to the environment of the womb. There is plenty going on – the baby is testing out the limits of its world, kicking, sucking its thumb, listening and busy getting on with growing. Amniotic fluid cushions the baby from impact; life is one long, warm feed, along with the comfort of the mother's heartbeat.

There are occasional disturbances to the well-being of the baby in the womb: the highly anxious mother whose adrenaline is flooding the baby's circulation; the baby hearing angry exchanges going on outside; the mother falling ill. Despite all this, most babies reach full term physically healthy, ready and prepared for the life that awaits.

Then comes the trauma of birth, which leaves indelible traces in the psyche of the infant.[1] The comfort of the womb is exchanged for almost heart-stopping compression as the birth process gets under way. Paediatricians refer to foetal distress when the oxygen supply to the baby is seriously compromised, but every baby passes through a rite of passage in which the forces of life and death are pitted one against the other. The terrors of the birth canal are only assuaged when the newborn infant is held in the arms of its mother, feeling the softness of her skin, taking in her smell and tasting the sweetness of her milk.

First Encounters with Loss

Nature has infinite wisdom in how things should be arranged, provided we do not mess it up with dogmatic and largely fashionable opinions as

---

1. For an account of how perinatal trauma may influence subsequent emotional development, see Grof (1985).

to what is 'good for the child'. The paediatrician Dr Truby King,[2] who was regarded in his time as a great authority on child care, pronounced that mothers should not go to their babies, no matter how much the baby cried, except for the four-hourly feed (and never at night). King taught that babies needed to be trained to be 'independent', a heartless regime that caused untold harm to many thousands of babies, some of whom suffer the consequences of disrupted emotional bonding to this day.

All severe privations of childhood leave their mark and an infant can only respond to overwhelming loss in one of three ways – taking refuge in withdrawal, becoming clinging, or learning how to survive without any deep attachments, a path that can lead to psychopathic behaviour later in life.[3]

In contrast, the toddler with healthy and confident attachment to its mother can risk losing sight of her for a time, not least out of sheer curiosity to explore the world, even just venturing into an adjacent room. When something frightening happens, real or imagined, the child runs back to the safety of its mother. Similarly, losing the comfort of breast milk is more than compensated for by the excitement of tasting different foods. Childhood at best is a great adventure, and bestowing confidence and security on their child is the indelible hallmark of good parenting.

Then comes the challenge of the wider social world. Every young person will feel frightened at times – the ego defences of fight or flight are built into all of us to deal with threats to our safety, be it physical or emotional.[4] The first day at school remains etched into most people's memory. The child is no longer at the epicentre of their social world. This big loss can be managed if kindly teachers step in to help, there are friends to be made and the lessons are fun. Then the child goes home with pride in a new accomplishment. Unfortunately, it is not always such a happy initiation and school phobia remains a major problem for child psychiatry services.

I am suggesting not only that loss is built into the blueprint of life, but also that in the right measure, losing what we count as safe and familiar can be the spur to growth. It holds true for that first day at school, or when the young adult falls in love and risks the pain of rejection, or when someone must face a life-threatening illness, or when

---

2. King (1942).
3. Bowlby (2005).
4. Such anxieties are not to be confused with the hypersensitivity that results from deep insecurity, leading either to withdrawal or compensatory grandiosity.

the person whose career falls apart finds a new path in life and salvages victory from defeat.

The Neurophysiology of Emotion

The mind is not reducible to the brain, but it certainly cannot do without it. Take the fight/flight response mentioned earlier. When an external threat is perceived, the brain tells the adrenal glands to release adrenaline in preparation for action. Importantly, the same physiological response can be triggered by something imagined, so that the insecure child, for example, who cannot cope with the absence of its mother, becomes highly anxious for fear of abandonment. In contrast, circulating endorphins, which are opioid peptides produced by the pituitary gland and hypothalamus in the brain, induce an immediate feeling of calm and well-being. Nature makes us this gift in the first few hours of life, when endorphins reach peak levels in the mother's bloodstream during labour and are imbibed by the baby in its first feed, thereby facilitating the bonding between them.

The centre for emotion in the central nervous system is located in specialised neural structures in the white matter of the brain known as the limbic system. This system mediates the emotional responses common to all mammals; for example, removal of the amygdala nucleus leads to passivity, while its stimulation – as may happen with epilepsy – can cause aggression.

Since the appearance of *Homo habilis* some 2 million years ago, the mass of the brain has greatly increased and the limbic system is now buried beneath the neocortex or grey matter, comprising the frontal lobes, the seat of reason and empathy.

The problem for humankind lies in the way the limbic system and the neocortex are liable to function – somewhat independently, and sometimes at odds with each other. This evolutionary quirk makes humanity vulnerable to the vicissitudes of human behaviour. In the case of the well-functioning human ego, reason and emotion are able to work together and serve us faithfully, enabling us to love, to bond and, through facing the many challenges of emotional conflict, to grow in maturity. When under threat, however, the limbic brain takes over and, as human history has shown, *Homo sapiens* is a species capable of destroying anyone or anything felt to be a threat to its survival. In earlier times, this served to protect tribal and national identities. These days, weapons technology and the global military industry cast a shadow over the survival of life on this planet.

The world now holds the prospect of catastrophic loss too unbearable for most people to contemplate. Instead, a dazzling array of electronic devices fills every waking hour, a constant stream of sensory impressions that leave little time or space for reflection.

Life without Soul

I have intimated that suffering is to be found in the blueprint of life. Moreover, when bearing with suffering, great or small, it has always been important to be able to turn to a more inclusive vision of life than that of one's own individual self – for example, the welfare and survival of kith and kin, giving shelter to those in need and working for the betterment of humanity. At the same time, the 'developed' world today is in the grip of a relentlessly materialist culture that stimulates and feeds the appetite of the consumer without encouraging human beings to look for deeper meaning and purpose, to reflect on the precious gift of life or to ask what life is for and how we may best play our part.

I see these deficiencies as reflecting a loss of soul in the post-modern secular world. If true, it also means that to treat disturbances of mind and body without reference to the soul is a serious omission.

With the word 'soul', I am describing the unique spiritual core of every human being. As atheists and humanists avow, this does not have to mean the survival of consciousness after bodily death. Some people look no further than the compass of their earthly lifetime for what they need to find, learn and experience. Others would rather trust in Providence not only for the life now, but also for the life hereafter.

In the West, the intellectual schism between materialist science and metaphysics has widened over the past 300 years. The dominant world-view of modernity is that we live in a fortuitous, mechanical universe. Karl Marx called religion the opium of the masses[5] and Sigmund Freud described it as a universal obsessional ritual and a mass delusion.[6] Despite such pronouncements, surveys have shown that over three-quarters of the UK population continue to believe in God or a Higher Presence,[7] most holding the view that the soul – the indestructible essence of each person – transcends the temporal bounds of birth and death.

---

5. Marx (1977: 131).
6. Freud (1907: 127).
7. See also *Whither the Soul of Psychiatry?*, this volume.

The Existential Void

When people turn away from the distractions of consumerism and question what life is really for, there is often uncertainty and unease. Now as always, parents wish for their children to be well, happy and successful. Friendships are the mainstay for many. Others hope the work that they do will contribute in some small way to human progress. However, when loss arises, whether through bereavement, breakdown of relationships, failure to make a success of one's work or loss of the dreamed-for future, spiritual values and beliefs may be called upon for the first time. Without an overarching sense of meaning and purpose – historically provided by the religious traditions – there may be nothing in the daily round to help sustain a person in the face of loss.

The life instinct is the foundation of the human ego and it is a powerful force. Small wonder, therefore, that many psychiatrists regard suicidal thinking as a symptom of depressive disorder, for the diagnosis purports to explain the anguish that drives a person to ask, 'What is the point in going on any longer?' or to announce, 'I am a failure', 'Nothing matters any more', 'There is no light, only darkness'.

In the face of such overwhelming misery, making the right diagnosis is crucial. Severe clinical depression, which can result in suicide, may require urgent and life-saving intervention, in which case the psychiatrist's role is unambiguously medical, and treatment follows accordingly. However, for the patient whose depression is symptomatic of a deep spiritual crisis, the situation is more complex. Apart from the clinician having to bear with diagnostic uncertainty, less than one-third of psychiatrists hold a spiritual or religious outlook. Most subscribe to a physicalist world-view, and this can lead to communication problems with the patient for whom the spiritual dimension is important.

To help someone through a spiritual crisis, the psychiatrist needs to show openness, empathy and genuine interest, coupled with a wide frame of reference. Above all, the psychiatrist should respect and support a person's spiritual enquiry. This does not mean having to provide answers, but it does mean encouraging the patient to ask those soul-searching questions of themselves and to look for the deepest heartfelt response from within. The psychiatrist needs to trust that those answers can and will be found when the patient is helped to seek out their own innate wisdom by paying attention to what the soul has to say.

Befriending the Ego

Barely has adulthood been reached before the ego is faced with alarming intimations of its own decline and eventual demise. Increasingly, the certain knowledge of ageing and death compels us to relinquish the cherished dreams of yesterday in favour of the stark truth that we do not – and cannot – have control over much of what is going to happen to us. From the perspective of the ego, it would seem that after making a good start, we are destined for a miserable end.

Everyone wants to be happy, but happiness can never be promised. Neither is it something that can be bought or borrowed. If our ego defences could yield gracefully before the inevitability of loss, we could be consoled in the knowledge of the greater gain – to have contributed to life, to the welfare of others and to have advanced one's soul as best one can along the way. Although our intellect may see the truth in this, the limbic brain resists. Worse still, where the emotions of fight and flight have not been moderated by love, the world is readily experienced as a hostile and dangerous place, out to strip the ego of its hard-won acquisitions. The resulting behaviour is fear-driven, the ego responding with arrogance, distrust and manipulation.

Such negative attributes have led to some spiritual traditions treating the ego as needing to be subjugated at all costs. Yet just as a knife can be used to kill or cut bread, the ego equally can be a force for good or ill. The difference lies between defensive patterns of behaviour based on fear and being open to new experiences based on co-operation, goodwill and trust.

When a person has been raised in a loving environment, the self, having felt itself to be loved, has love to give. The precept 'Love your neighbour as yourself'[8] arises naturally. Whereas the psychology of fear treats love as a commodity that must be bought, borrowed or stolen, the psychology of love is one of abundance, based on the axiom that 'what goes around comes around'. It follows that to feed others is to feed oneself.

Feeling both loving and loved engenders compassion, and with it, forgiveness for others and for oneself. From time to time, the ego can be expected to resort to its old ways, prompting us to act hurtfully or thoughtlessly. Nevertheless, love does not require us to be perfect, only to be capable of remorse and a willingness to try one's best. Moreover, the recognition that everyone struggles alike is a great spur to humility. When the self is loved, the ego lowers its defences and can begin to see

---

8. Matthew 22:39. *The Holy Bible*, NIV.

the bigger picture – that it is part of a greater whole. 'I' and 'mine' widens to 'we' and 'ours'. This is the opening to spirituality: the realisation that 'I belong to more than myself'.

Society at large inevitably mirrors the emotional life of the human family. At this stage in the evolution of our species, the future of humankind lies in the balance, for we are still susceptible to the fight/flight response of the ego under threat. To stop fighting and start making common cause, humanity urgently needs to start listening to the soul.

Suffering, East and West

I referred earlier to the spiritual practice of attempting to subjugate the ego. Since the ego will always fight back, this frequently brings about further suffering. It seems to me more helpful to take the ego by the hand, so to speak, and spend time instructing it in the way of the soul – for the ego is not ineducable. I like to picture the influence of the soul on the ego along the lines of a good parent dealing with a headstrong child. As the ego begins to attune to the soul perspective, its agitation subsides, it becomes more peaceful and its energies can be put to better use.[9] However, such a 'child' needs understanding, patience and love.

It is no coincidence that the study of mental disorder flourished in the West, for since the time of the Renaissance we have been fascinated by the complexity of the individual psyche. In the East, there is a more pragmatic tradition, one of setting aside the burdensome contents of the psyche while aiming to purify heart and mind through meditation. This has led to important East–West cultural differences towards the negative, or shadow, aspect of the self.

Buddhists and Hindus concentrate on 'right conduct' and the development of wisdom that will influence successive earthly incarnations according to the law of karma.[10] Desire and attachment are treated as the inevitable cause of suffering. Thus, abstaining from desire – which leads naturally to letting go of attachment – will end suffering and free a person from the bonds of karma, expediting release

---

9. Just as a child brings new experiences, challenges and learning to its parent, the soul likewise benefits from its relationship with the ego, whether for the duration of a single life or, as Eastern religions teach, over many lifetimes.
10. The law of karma teaches that cause brings about effect, which in turn becomes the next cause. Far from suggesting fatalism, knowledge of karma reminds a person that their destiny, for good or ill, lies in their own hands.

from the cycle of incarnation and thereby bringing the ultimate peace and bliss of nirvana.

Taoism, rooted in ancient China, is unique in holding that there is no such intrinsic thing as badness; suffering is the manifestation of the imbalance of *yin* and *yang*, and when the rhythms of Nature and life are truly understood and observed, harmony spontaneously arises.[11]

Neither karma nor the rhythms of Nature feature in the Abrahamic faiths. Instead, emphasis is given to repentance of one's sins. In Judaism, Maimonides' *Rules of Repentance* in the Mishneh Torah and *The Gates of Repentance*, by Rabbenu Yonah of Gerona, set out in detail the exacting requirements of true repentance. In Islam, the Koran states that repentance is the most noble and beloved form of obedience in the eyes of Allah.

In Christian doctrine, suffering is seen as both a test of faith and a path to redemption. In atoning for the sins of humanity, Jesus makes the supreme sacrifice. Yet Jesus himself cries out on the cross, *Eli, Eli, lema sabachthani* ('My God, my God, why have you forsaken me')[12] before breathing his last with the words, 'Father, into your hands I commit my spirit'.[13] For Christians, the crucifixion offers a guiding light through the dark night of the soul, with the promise of redemption in the embrace of God's love.

Psychotherapists are less concerned with sin than guilt. Some people are prone to a disproportionate sense of guilt and suffer accordingly. Others avoid finding fault with themselves and would rather blame others. Jung saw this latter human tendency as a potential threat to the future of humanity. He held that the shadow side of the personality must be recognised and integrated if humankind is to stop projecting the shadow on to others and then attacking it there. In his words: 'Everyone carries a shadow, and the less it is embodied in the individual's conscious life, the blacker and denser it is'.[14]

Individual and Collective Suffering

When we wrestle with the question of suffering, asking what we have done to deserve it or what kind of God allows it (as atheists like to point out), we often find ourselves going round in circles. Yet from

---

11. The classic Taoist text is the *Tao Te Ching*, attributed to Lao Tsu in the 6th century BCE. See Feng & English (1973).
12. Matthew 27:46. *The Holy Bible*, NIV.
13. Luke 23:46. *The Holy Bible*, NIV.
14. Jung (1938: 76).

a transpersonal perspective, such an enquiry can be rewarding, since it allows for the possibility that through adversity the soul grows in understanding, wisdom and compassion.[15]

Moreover, it has been suggested that one person's suffering may be in the service of helping others awaken to the spiritual values of caring and concern. In this sense, the torture and execution to which Jesus submitted can be seen as a supreme sacrifice made to awaken the conscience of the world. This highlights the ambiguous status of psychiatry today, for had Pontius Pilate been able to order a psychiatric examination, imagine what may have followed; instead of crucifixion, compulsory treatment for a delusional disorder! Further, before we dismiss Judas Iscariot as a bad character, we must remember that without him, 'the law and the prophets' could not have been fulfilled. Is it right to condemn Judas? Possibly, he was entrusted with the most difficult task of all the disciples.

Although karma may be rooted in the behaviour of the individual, collective karma is no less important. Genocide is a shocking crime against humanity and far from ending with the Holocaust, it has tragically continued since, in Biafra, Uganda, Cambodia, Rwanda, the Balkans and Iraq, Syria and now Myanmar. How else to break the cycle of persecution except through forgiveness?

Why Should We Forgive?

For most of us, forgiveness does not come easy. Yet without forgiveness, a person can remain imprisoned in feelings of hurt, anger, bitterness and often guilt that can last a lifetime – some would say, many lifetimes.

Moreover, if our species is not to destroy itself, finding the capacity to forgive is going to be pivotal to the future of humankind. Can we make use of the many and deep wounds of life to help raise the consciousness of our world to a new level? This requires us to hold a larger view of humanity than that comprehended by the ego.

Since the ego is governed by self-survival and knows no other life than this one, its instinct when threatened, far from being forgiving, is retaliatory. In contrast, the soul tells a different story. Since it transcends the body, the soul is unconcerned with physical survival, holds

---

15. It has been said that from the soul perspective, however great the misfortune, there is no such thing as a 'bad' experience. Given the anguish and suffering endured by many people, it is important to clarify that a distinction is being made here between human experience and the life of the (eternal) soul.

no resentments and views the comings and goings of life with equanimity. It is in the original nature of the soul to want nothing more than for the incarnated self to outgrow the narrow concerns of the ego and become conscious of the sacred oneness of life.

In my work as a psychiatrist, I have been struck by the painful and unforeseen challenges that it seems everyone sooner or later must encounter. Invariably, we are confronted with what we most need to face, which surprisingly often turns out to be a lesson in forgiveness – whether of ourselves or others. Learning to forgive opens the way to wholeness and healing.

To begin with, the ego knows nothing about healing, being occupied with ambition and self-interest. Yet in a world driven by the needs of the ego, every human being will, intentionally or not, inflict and receive, pain. Throughout the turbulent business of life, the soul brings its influence to bear on the ego. The ego may be slow to learn, but the soul is a patient teacher. Importantly, the ego discovers that love is not a personal possession, but a universal gift to be shared.

This brings the ego to its greatest challenge – finding love not just for oneself and one's kith and kin, but for those who have badly hurt us. The author Immaculee Ilibagiza, whose entire family was slaughtered in the Rwandan holocaust, gives an inspiring account.[16] In the midst of her terrible grief, she came to recognise through prayer that the man who single-handedly had murdered her family was a child of God as much as she, and face-to-face she was able to forgive him.

Forgiveness is the supreme test of love. Jesus spelled it out like this: '…love your enemies and pray for those who persecute you, that you may be children of your Father in heaven'.[17] Just as the lotus, symbol of transformation, cannot flower without its roots in the mud, the soul finds an opportunity for forgiveness in every hurt given and received.

Desirable though it may be, a person cannot always bring themselves to forgive, and it is not for anyone to insist upon it. Nevertheless, what I have generally found is that a person would *wish* to be able to forgive, if it only felt possible. This is because despite the wounds of the ego, the soul impulse cannot be killed off. The unforgiving heart yearns for freedom from its chains and once we make contact with the wish to forgive, we start out on a journey of love in which we too can be forgiven, find redemption and make our return to the Garden of Eden; no longer a place of innocence but a place of wisdom.

---

16. Ilibagiza (2006).
17. Matthew 5:44–45. *The Holy Bible*, NIV.

References

Bowlby, J. (2005) *The Making and Breaking of Affectional Bonds*. Routledge Classics.
Feng, G.F. & English, J. (trans.) (1973) *Lao Tsu: Tao Te Ching*. Wildwood House.
Freud, S. (1907) Obsessive actions and religious practices. Reprinted [1959] in *The Standard Edition of the Complete Psychological Works of Sigmund Freud*, vol. 9 (trans. & ed. J. Strachey). Hogarth Press.
Grof, S. (1985) *Beyond the Brain*. State University of New York Press.
Ilibagiza, I. (2006) *Left to Tell*. Hay House.
Jung, C.G. (1938) Psychology and religion. Reprinted [1958] in *C.G. Jung: The Collected Works*, vol. 11, Psychology and Religion: West and East (eds H. Read, M. Fordham & G. Adler). Routledge and Kegan Paul.
King, F.T. (1942) *Feeding and Care of Baby*. Macmillan and Co.
Marx, K. (1977) *Critique of Hegel's Philosophy of Right*. Cambridge University Press.

3

Spirituality and Psychiatry – Crossing the Divide

'A fish said to another fish, "Above this sea of ours there is another sea, with creatures swimming in it – and they live there, even as we live here." The fish replied, "Pure fancy! When you know that everything that leaves our sea by even an inch, and stays out of it, dies. What proof have you of other lives in other seas?"' [1]

I would like to say something about how I came to be involved in the field of spirituality in mental healthcare. I want to do so not because I think there is anything special about my case, but because it may encourage others in the healthcare professions to feel they can do the same. Although prejudice against spirituality is still encountered in some quarters, in recent years there has been an appreciable shift of opinion, enough to ensure that health professionals who declare their interest in the spiritual dimension will find themselves in good company.

After qualifying as a doctor in 1969 but before specialising in psychiatry, I worked for 2 years in acute hospital medicine. The experience lives vividly with me to this day. The technology of coronary care had just arrived, along with a whole raft of advances in the investigation and treatment of a wide range of diseases. The medical model was mechanistic through and through, as it remains to this day.

Coming up with a diagnosis leading to a treatment that is specific and effective offers a great deal of intellectual satisfaction for the doctor, as well as the pleasure of seeing one's patient get better. I confess that I was rather less taken with the task of supporting patients with

First published as chapter in *Spirituality, Values and Mental Health* (eds E. Coyte, P. Gilbert & V. Nicholls), pp. 161–171. © 2007 Jessica Kingsley. Reproduced with permission.

---

1. Gibran (1963: 45).

chronic conditions, unlikely to recover and at best being maintained in status quo. There seemed to be less 'to do' and no one helped young doctors understand the art of 'being with'.

In those days, medical students learned to dissect dead bodies long before they were ever allowed to touch a live patient. Later, when doing our obstetrics, we helped deliver babies under the watchful eye of the midwife. Even so, the miracle of birth took second place to the need to examine the baby, check for genetic abnormalities, listen to the heart and so on. I remember a few years later trying to resuscitate a baby in casualty. It was a cot death and there was nothing we were able to do. I had to tell the mother. She was inconsolable, of course, and I felt wretched too. I could not think of what to say. Death, whether in the young or old, was invariably the great enemy of Life, and we had lost the battle.

I am not arguing against medical technology. I needed a heart valve replacement some years back, without which I would certainly have died. Nevertheless, in recalling my early years as a doctor, I am aware of the difficulty I had in finding the confidence and the time to relate to the person rather than the disease.

Communication skills have now become part of the medical school curriculum but enormous problems remain. Young doctors still feel there should be an answer to every question. It is not easy to say, 'I don't know'. Firstly, such an admission is not what the patient wants to hear. Secondly, it puts the doctor in the less assured position of being a fellow traveller on the unpredictable journey of life. The patient has to tolerate the pain of uncertainty, while the doctor, whose role helps relieve him of personal anxiety of illness and death by naming the problem firmly in the 'other', may both feel and be perceived as more vulnerable.

Nevertheless, a doctor who joins forces with the patient by reaching out to the patient's fear and pain is opening the way for the medicine of healing, of 'making whole'. Feeling whole does not promise cure, but it enables a person to make the best possible recovery and, when illness cannot be relieved, to continue life with an intact sense of meaning and purpose.

At this juncture I would like to say something about spirituality. The word has been variously defined and I understand it to be about both *being* and *doing*. Spirituality is the experience of deeply felt meaning and purpose in life and a sense of wholeness and belonging that brings harmony and peace. For some, this finds fulfilment in loving human relationships, while for others it must admit the relationship with God as the ultimate source of love. As a transpersonal quest, spirituality entails searching for answers about the infinite that lies beyond earthly life, and can be particularly important at times of illness, loss, bereavement and death.

To see why our medical care has become so devoid of spirituality and so very mechanistic in orientation, we need to understand its roots in the Newtonian science of the past 300 years. It happens that Isaac Newton was both a great empirical scientist and a deeply religious man, but his researches into the properties of physical matter were taken by his successors to mean that God as the prime mover had to be located elsewhere, beyond a mechanistic universe. Such a remote God could hardly be expected to influence the workings of the human body except by means of occasional, miraculous (inexplicable) healing.

By the end of the 19th century, disease had become identified with organ pathology, and the subsequent discovery of bacterial infections, biochemical, degenerative and congenital disorders, cancer and other conditions all reinforced the materialist perspective. God was dismissed by science as irrelevant, with the Church ousted from medical care except for providing comfort, offering spiritual guidance to the afflicted and administering the last rites.

Psychiatry as Science of the Mind

Psychiatry as a science is rooted in 19th-century European neurology, with the same emphasis on the physical basis of disease. For example, neurosyphilis had been demonstrated to cause mental changes resulting from damage to the brain, while porphyria and vitamin deficiencies were shown to affect mental functioning. Emil Kraepelin classified severe mental illness into schizophrenia and manic depressive (bipolar) disorder, thereby reinforcing the concept of distinct categories of mental disorder.[2]

Major mental illness does indeed respond to some extent to pharmacological treatments, although the causes remain unknown. Unfortunately, this has led many psychiatrists to treat the numerous and varied disturbances of mood and thought they routinely see in clinic as diagnostic of mental disorder requiring medication. General practice likewise has been influenced by this climate of opinion. All too often, the prescription serves a ritual function, a poor substitute for time needed by patients to talk, be heard and feel understood.

---

2. Kraepelin's dichotomous classification is now regarded as increasingly suspect. See Craddock & Owen (2005).

What about Sigmund Freud's remarkable contribution to the study of the mind? Freud's early belief that neurosis would similarly prove to be founded in brain dysfunction never materialised. Instead, psychoanalysis has run for a hundred years parallel to mainstream psychiatry. Freud's epic approach to the study of the psyche elegantly charts the conscious and unconscious reaches of the human mind, but it simply has not worked for serious mental illness.

Many mental health services today offer a range of symptom-orientated psychological therapies as well as medication. Psychoanalysis undoubtedly paved the way for shorter-term psychodynamic treatments. Behavioural psychology has led to cognitive–behavioural therapies, while family therapy is based largely on systems theory. Yet with the exception of the transpersonal approach, to which I shall come later, such therapies rarely stray beyond the pragmatics of everyday life. The big questions about birth, life and death that so often occupy the troubled mind generally get no chance of being heard. Yet we know that such concerns will frequently be voiced by patients, if only the psychiatrist shows interest.

In drawing attention to the history that shaped Western science, I have painted a picture of medicine, and psychiatry too, somewhat lacking in warmth. Of course, there are countless physicians and surgeons who intuitively and compassionately care for the 'whole person'. However, the reductive-analytic approach of Western science has led to a dazzling proliferation of specialisms, with the danger that the part is minutely examined while the whole person never gets seen.

My training in hospital medicine came at the end of the era of consultant physicians who were expected to know just about everything. Rather naively, I expected psychiatrists to be equally well informed. Moving to the renowned Maudsley Hospital and Institute of Psychiatry in London, I was struck by how the mind was considered in isolation, as entirely separate from the body. Liaison psychiatry was in its infancy and more or less confined to seeing patients with overdoses admitted to King's College Hospital across the road, or unexpected cases of delirium tremens on the medical and surgical wards. Psychosomatic medicine, too, seemed to have run out of steam – all this being prior to the discovery of psychoneuroimmunology.

At the Maudsley, we earnestly debated the finer points of diagnosis much along the same lines as in general medicine. Yet this seemed to be more about gleaning intellectual satisfaction from the work than having much bearing on management and treatment. The clinical environment felt very impersonal; patients were talked *about* more than they were talked *with*. Psychiatry seemed to have no soul, although at the time it would not have occurred to me to put it that way. I found myself drawn to psychoanalysis. Aside from personal issues that I wanted to explore, the Maudsley Hospital psychotherapy department was the one place where time was given to 'be with' one's patient and I soon realised that this was what I had come into psychiatry for.

The Search for Soul

Psychoanalysis took up a lot of my time over the next few years. Sigmund Freud had an answer for just about everything that lay between birth and death, and it all made good sense. My intellect was fired and my admiration for Freud was unbounded. The training and the clinical work went well and later I went on to specialise in group analysis. I worked hard and became a consultant, and I would like to think I helped a fair number of patients. Later I came to see that Freud had been for me an irresistible father figure and had I remained an obedient son, I would never have left home and made my own way in the world.

The work of Carl Jung barely got a mention at the Maudsley and I wondered why, until I read about his exile by Freud. Visiting Freud's house in Vienna, where the walls are lined with hundreds of photographs of Freud, his family, friends and colleagues, I noticed that there was not a single picture of Jung, the disciple Freud had marked out as his natural successor. My curiosity aroused, I started to read Jung and I found myself engaged with a mind as profound as Freud's, with one great difference. Jung sought to understand Man not only as the product of his childhood, but also as endowed with an ineluctable spiritual birthright.

This opened a new door for me. Patients had not infrequently brought to me what I would these days call spiritual concerns – deep, searching questions about the whole meaning and purpose of life, especially of suffering. I had been inclined to interpret these in relation to problems encountered in childhood and in subsequent relationships difficulties, and I was not always wrong. Yet sometimes I knew I had missed something vital, and it was no good ascribing it to 'resistance' on the part of the patient. I began to think that my need for an all-explanatory psychology of humankind was serving to shield me (and sometimes my patient) from the unknown, not the 'small' unknown of the human unconscious mind, but the greater unknown that goes way beyond birth and death.

Around this time, I was introduced to psychodrama by Marcia Karp, who had personally trained with Jacob Moreno.[3] To my surprise, this therapeutic approach found places in me that psychoanalysis had never reached. Memories, dreams and reflections of my own erupted with full force, and could be dramatised without the constraint of having to sit or lie down (the golden rule of analytical therapy). The effect was to connect body with mind and to discover that the body has memories of its own, even before birth. Taking the cue from psychodrama, I was emboldened to approach life with greater emotional freedom and spontaneity than I had found in the world of psychoanalysis.

I also saw how psychodrama can reveal the workings of the soul, as I discovered in one of the first sessions I attended:

> Ruth had been deeply embittered by the loss of her son some years before. In the session, she was encouraged to revisit the roadside scene of the car crash in which he had been killed. Weeping in despair, she cried out 'God, why have you done this to me'. The psychodrama therapist instantly directed her to reverse roles with God. At once, this mother's face changed, becoming calm and composed, her sobbing ceased and [as God] she said with immense dignity, 'I have done nothing to you. Your son chose to die, so that he would not suffer any more. Be happy for him, and thankful for his life that brought you joy.'

Ruth was amazed by what had come out of her own mouth. She saw the meaning of it perfectly and for the first time since her son's death, she could begin to heal.[4]

I have detailed this event because it was a defining moment for me. I perceived that the soul is a reservoir of deep wisdom with the power to overcome the most painful of life's traumas.

I began to question the limitations of psychodynamic psychotherapy. For instance, therapists talk a great deal about projection and splitting as defences against psychic pain, while entrusting recovery to the resolution of the transference by way of interpretation.[5] The psychological frame of reference is that of child and parent, the therapist

---

3. Jacob L. Moreno (1889–1974), psychiatrist, sociologist and the founder of psychodrama.
4. Also cited in *Soul-Centred Psychotherapy*, this volume.
5. The analytical method encourages the emergence of unresolved childhood emotions, which are unconsciously projected on to the therapist (a process called transference). The therapist remains as neutral as possible in order to be a 'blank screen' for such projections. By means of interpretation, the therapist endeavours to help the patient understand what is happening and to own such feelings instead of splitting them off and projecting them on to the therapist and others. The process is often painful and good 'parenting' is required on the part of the therapist to enable the patient to feel sufficiently secure to cope with what is going on.

offering what has been called 'the corrective emotional experience'. Standing *in loco parentis* is no small undertaking, on top of which the dependency needs of the patient frequently result in the therapist being experienced as omnipotent, patently a God-like role. But what about a patient's deepest and most heartfelt questions? 'Why am I here? What is it all for? What happens when I die? Why must I suffer?' Most therapists will avoid discussion in order to preserve the status of the transference or, if necessary, will take these fundamental existential concerns as problems arising from unconscious and unresolved childhood conflicts.

Healing and Wholeness[6]

At around this time, I came to know a number of healers, and I was struck by the good results they were having across a range of physical and emotional conditions. I decided to learn more and applied to train at the College of Healing, where I first met 'intuitives', who could directly perceive the human energy field or *aura*. From a medical point of view, any therapeutic effect from hands-on healing is attributed to suggestibility (placebo effect). But what if the 'energies' being employed are real, although beyond the instrumentation of current science to detect?

There is now good empirical evidence, based on a large number of randomised controlled trials, that healing works.[7] As to how, it has been suggested that quantum entanglement may hold the key.[8] Indeed, some quantum physicists argue that matter has (cosmic) intelligence inscribed in its very substance and that consciousness itself is a non-local unified field in which we are all immersed.[9]

Such a cosmology describes a participative spiritual universe, fundamentally conscious in design, and very possibly evolving so as to know more of itself! The implications of holographic cosmology are profound – that the fundamental processes of life on our little planet are homologous with life throughout the length and breadth of the cosmos, while at the same time our human capacity for love – the essence of which is connection – similarly reflects the oneness of all that is.[10]

We generally take the world of our ordinary sense perception for granted; after all, it comprises the 'consensus reality' of everyday life.

---

6. Healing and wholeness share the same root, both words deriving from *hal*, *hel* or *heil* in Saxon, High German or Old Norse respectively.
7. For an extensive review of controlled studies on healing, see Benor (2002).
8. Radin (2006).
9. Goswami (1993).
10. For a general introduction, see Talbot (1996).

However, I began to question whether there is any such thing as reality in and of itself, for what and how a person perceives will depend on their subjective disposition. Most of us see and hear things the same way (in line with what quantum physicists call the collapse of the probability wave). Yet it is not always so, as the accumulated body of research into paranormal phenomena now demonstrates.

This raises another difficulty for psychiatry, for how then should we distinguish between mental illness and paranormal experiences, not least between psychosis and spiritual crisis? To make matters more complicated, there can be an overlap between the two.

One way is to postpone making a judgement about the status of a symptom while exploring what value it holds for the person and whether it stands to help the person find a more meaningful and purposeful life. Breakdown may yet turn into breakthrough.

This takes us away from the notion of disease, which is an objective measure, to that of illness, a subjective measure of the impact of physical or emotional adversity on a person. In this sense, a person can be 'well' in themselves even as they are dying, finding wholeness of being and fulfilment in the moment – a sober reminder to those of us who overlook the precious 'now' and instead worry about a future that must, in any case, eventually bring death our way.

The life instinct is a strong one and the promise of cure is, of course, welcome news. It restores, in the short term, a sense of immortality that distances us from the day of reckoning. However, while death has aptly been described as the one appointment no one is in a hurry to keep, the materialist world-view of our time makes the ending of life, including the loss of loved ones, a tragic and irreparable parting of the ways.

Death as Transition

The death of someone close can precipitate breakdown in an already vulnerable person. Yet the belief that consciousness ends with death is a modern myth propagated by a culture of material realism. Importantly, we can appreciate the achievements of 300 years of science without succumbing to its physicalist ideology. In any event, there continues to be intense speculation about life after death and the majority of people continue to believe in an afterlife.[11]

---

11. A 2008 UK survey by Theos showed that 53% of the population believe in life after death, 55% believe in heaven and 70% believe in the human soul (Spencer & Weldin, 2012). These figures compare interestingly with Geoffrey Gorer's

Mindful of this, the spiritually informed psychiatrist sets out to help a person value, trust and explore the authenticity of their own experience as fully as they can. No counter-culture proselytising is called for; this would be to replace one kind of conditioning with another. Fortunately, since our innate archetypes remain alive and well, it is only necessary to ask with genuine interest what a person would hope to be possible and to invite the telling of that story.

For example, when a bereaved patient entreats 'if only my mum were still here', it may be helpful to proceed by finding out what he[12] is wishing he could ask or say, and then to encourage him to take the opportunity to talk with 'mum'. This can be done simply by asking him to close his eyes, to imagine her there in the room, and to go right ahead and speak with her. When he has done so, the patient is asked to sit for a minute longer, eyes closed, and listen to, or simply experience, what may come back. Sometimes it is a verbal response, or it may be a silent embrace. Crucial unfinished business can be completed this way, often with the farewell that had not been possible in life. It is not unusual for the person to have had a profound sense of the presence of the deceased, and sometimes actually to have seen or heard them.

While it is generally acknowledged that in cases of bereavement, spontaneous sightings of the deceased individual can occur, what is less often recognised is just how frequently they happen. In one study of widows, 14% reported a visual hallucination of their deceased spouse, and nearly a half described experiencing a sense of 'presence'.[13]

Here is an example of working transpersonally with bereavement that calls for no special training on the part of the therapist other than empathy and imagination:

> My patient Gareth was referred by his general practitioner for depression. He had cared for his mother during her illness with cancer and after she died he was burdened with the memory of her suffering.
>
> When Gareth came for the second session, he said something had happened that had been a shock. One night, soon after lying down, he had clearly seen his mother standing at the end of the bed. When he rubbed his eyes and looked again, she had gone. He thought he must be going out of his mind.
>
> Rather than simply explaining to Gareth that such hallucinations can happen and that he shouldn't worry about it, I asked him to recall

---

  1955 study *Exploring English Character*, in which only 47% of people reported belief in the afterlife (Gorer, 1955: 253).
12. The male gender is denoted here, without prejudice, to refer to both male and female.
13. Rees (1971).

how his mother had looked. He said it was strange but she was smiling. Had she spoken? Gareth replied that nothing was said but he felt she was somehow telling him she was well and he shouldn't worry. I put to Gareth that this visit by his mother was not only nothing to be afraid of but also that it could be of great value and a comfort to him. Gareth said he was so relieved to think his mother, wherever she was, could feel well and happy again. His mood began to lift the same day.

What does this say about life after death? It says much or little, depending on your point of view. It can be understood on the psychological level, the spiritual level, or both. Either way, it breaks the terrifying finality of death because the mind has been helped to transcend the customary limits of space-time.

For some people, spirituality means finding the greatest depth of meaning and purpose in their existence without reference to 'other worlds'. In my own case, however, my studies led me to envisage the human soul as a scintilla of cosmic consciousness that incarnates in order to experience, learn and grow. I was curious to find out more about my own 'soul journey' and this took me to the study of 'past life' regression, in both theory and practice.

The Transpersonal Perspective

Anomalous perceptual experiences transgress the Newtonian rule set of space-time and thereby fly in the face of consensus reality. They are more likely to arise when a person is in an 'altered' state of consciousness, but this does not have to mean a state of trance or from taking a psychoactive drug. Subtle changes in consciousness take place in reverie, when the mind is stilled in meditation and prayer, in the hypnagogic state, or simply with therapeutic guidance. Here is an example:

> Michael came to see me for panic attacks triggered by a fear of suffocation. After taking a history that gave no other clue as to the cause, I invited Michael to close his eyes, to 'go into' that feeling of suffocation, then to 'look around' him and describe what is happening. Michael became visibly agitated and reported finding himself in a burning house. Unable to escape, the scene ended in his death by smoke inhalation, with Michael 'looking on' at his lifeless body. I encouraged him to 'let go' and Michael experienced floating peacefully away – much as reported by near-death experience survivors. Michael's fear and agitation having passed, I brought him back into the present with the vivid experience of having found release from the trauma of that death. Following the session, Michael's fear of suffocation was relieved and did not return.

Who is to say what has really happened here? Some would argue the case for 'past lives', while others would see it as therapeutic use of active imagination. From the clinical perspective, the important thing is that the treatment is effective.[14]

Once I had become used to working transpersonally beyond the bounds of space and time, I went on to study spirit release therapy, as described in this representative illustration:

> Abby, a woman in her mid-life, otherwise well and with no history of mental illness, described feeling strangely burdened by her mother's continuing 'presence'[15] in the family home since her death some months before. Abby explained that her mother used to suffer from depression, and the atmosphere in the house continued to feel oppressive, 'as if Mum had never left'. Noticing her words, I asked Abby about her beliefs regarding the soul and the afterlife. Abby did wonder if her mother was still suffering 'beyond the grave'. I suggested we might explore whether Abby's mother was finding it difficult to 'let go and move on', to which Abby readily agreed.
>
> I invited Abby to relax and let her mother 'speak' through her, allowing the words to come spontaneously. I then had a 'conversation' with the mother in which it turned out that she was afraid to leave the familiarity of home and the comfort of her daughter. I assured Abby's mother that when she moved on into the 'light' she would find love, acceptance and a new beginning. To help her on her way, I asked if she would like an angelic guide to join her. Mother could feel the guide gently take her by the hand, and together they walked into the light. At once, Abby's sense of oppression lifted – and was gone for good.[16]

Is this simply a way of externalising unresolved emotion? Is the patient improvising her mother's words based on her knowledge of family history? Could this indeed be engaging with another reality 'beyond the veil'? Moreover, do we as clinicians have to know the answer, provided the therapy is consonant with the patient's beliefs and leads to a good outcome?

Anomalous perceptions do not in themselves signify mental illness, as Gordon Claridge's work on schizotypy has clearly shown,[17] and given that at least 10% of the general population will have such a

---

14. See also *Past Life Memory – A Key to Understanding the Self?*, this volume.
15. William James, who studied the phenomenon of 'presence', wrote: 'it would appear to be an extremely definite and positive state of mind, coupled with a belief in the reality of its object quite as strong as any direct sensation ever gives. And yet no sensation seems to be connected with it at all' (1950: 322–323).
16. See also *The Contribution of Spirit Release Therapy to Mental Health*, this volume.
17. Claridge (1997).

perception during their lifetime,[18] the experience is clearly too common to be indicative of pathology.

I have described elsewhere[19] a number of case studies in which my aim is to engage with the existential reality of my patients' beliefs and perceptions rather than to objectify them. The approach is generally to see our lives as part of a greater, spiritual whole that encompasses and transcends material reality.

There are, however, provisos when working transpersonally. First, there must be diagnostic acumen when deciding on a transpersonal approach. Second, there are ethical considerations; it is important to be in tune with the patient's preferences and beliefs. Third, no interpretation should be imposed – let water find its own level. Fourth, we need to recognise that sometimes chaplaincy is best placed to help the troubled soul. Lastly, the spiritual must always be grounded in the psychological.

Psychiatrists who are open to the spiritual dimension – whether or not working transpersonally – will have the reward of touching the souls of their patients, just as their patients will likewise touch them, and both will surely feel the better for it.

In Conclusion

In psychiatric practice, treatment is largely pragmatic, based on the prevailing bio-psychosocial model of our times. As a working model it is widely endorsed, yet spirituality, the highest function of the imaginal mind, has got left out. This is something of an irony since psyche means spirit (or soul), and it is a lack that urgently needs putting right. Apart from the importance of encouraging patients to feel able fully to confide in their psychiatrists, research over the past 20 years has shown that spirituality is good for both mental and physical health.[20]

In this paper, I have given a short account of how, over the years, I found myself taking a spiritually orientated approach to mental healthcare. Every practitioner ends up working in their own preferred way and this has been mine. However, I have also wanted to convey that such an approach need not feel remote or esoteric. At the very least, a psychiatrist can easily include taking a spiritual history as part of the consultation process. Just a few questions asked with sincerity and

---

18. For studies of auditory and visual hallucinations in healthy (non-psychotic) adults, see the Julian Jaynes Society (2017).
19. *Soul-Centred Psychotherapy*, this volume.
20. See *Mental Health and Spirituality*, in Powell (2017).

interest will elicit a person's important beliefs, how they approach their problems, and whether they see the challenges of life as having a spiritual meaning. If a person is searching for answers that lie beyond the bounds of consensus reality, a transpersonal approach may be especially helpful. In any event, the practitioner who can be a caring confidant for their patients' soul-searching will be amply rewarded, for all that is required is to be fully 'present'. The soul in its wisdom will find the place of healing and it is our privilege to be able to help give it the occasion.

References

Benor, D.J. (2002) *Healing Research*, vol. 1, Spiritual Healing: Scientific Validation of a Healing Revolution. Vision Publications.
Claridge, G.A. (1997) *Schizotypy: Implications for Illness and Health*. Oxford University Press.
Craddock, N. & Owen, M. (2005) The beginning of the end for the Kraepelinian dichotomy. *British Journal of Psychiatry*, 186(5), 364–366.
Gibran, K. (1963) Other Seas. In *The Forerunner*. William Heinemann.
Gorer, G. (1955) *Exploring English Character*. Criterion Books.
Goswami, A. (1993) *The Self-Aware Universe*. Tarcher/Putnam.
James, W. (1950) *Principles of Psychology*, vol. 2. Dover Publications.
Julian Jaynes Society (2017) Auditory and visual hallucinations in normal (non-psychotic) adults. Available at: http://www.julianjaynes.org/supporting-evidence_auditory-hallucinations.php (accessed 11 July 2017).
Powell, A. (2017) *The Ways of the Soul. A Psychiatrist Reflects: Essays on Life, Death and Beyond*. Muswell Hill Press.
Radin, D. (2006) *Entangled Minds*. Paraview Pocket Books.
Rees, W.D. (1971) The hallucinations of widowhood. *BMJ*, 4, 37–41.
Spencer, N. & Weldin, H. (2012) *Post-religious Britain? The Faith of the Faithless*. Theos.
Talbot, M. (1996) *The Holographic Universe*. HarperCollins.

4

Whither the Soul of Psychiatry?

To understand the state of psychiatry today, and to see where it is most likely heading, I want to give some historical context, starting with the early history of spiritual and religious beliefs concerning mental well-being. I will then outline the growing dominance of the new world-view of science and how the fledgling profession of psychiatry made the secular mind its exclusive focus. Lastly, I want to highlight a growing recognition in recent years that patients' spiritual concerns can have profound implications for diagnosis, treatment and outcome.

Before embarking on this overview, and because there is often confusion about the difference between religion and spirituality, I will start with a useful distinction drawn by Harold Koenig:[1]

> 'Religion: an organised system of beliefs, practices, rituals, and symbols designed to facilitate closeness to the sacred or transcendent (God, higher power, or ultimate truth/reality).
>
> Spirituality: the personal quest for understanding answers to ultimate questions about life, about meaning, and about relationship with the sacred or transcendent, which may (or may not) lead to or arise from the development of religious rituals and the formation of community.'

The Royal College of Psychiatrists' Spirituality and Psychiatry Special Interest Group suggests the following:[2]

> 'Spirituality can be as broad as the essentially human, personal and interpersonal dimension, which integrates and transcends the cultural, religious, psychological, social and emotional aspects of the person, or more specifically concerned with "soul" or "spirit".'

Paper prepared for the 1st British Congress on Medicine and Spirituality, 'Furthering the Spiritual Dimension of Psychiatry in the United Kingdom', London, June 2007.

---

1. Koenig et al. (2001).
2. http://www.rcpsych.ac.uk/spirit

The spiritual dimension is strongly implied in a statement by the World Health Organization (WHO) that good medical practice should take account of a person's faith, beliefs and values in finding healing:[3]

> '...the health professions have largely followed a medical model, which seeks to treat patients by focusing on medicines and surgery, and gives less importance to beliefs and to faith – in healing, in the physician and in the doctor–patient relationship. This reductionism or mechanistic view of patients as being only a material body is no longer satisfactory. Patients and physicians have begun to realise the value of elements such as faith, hope and compassion in the healing process.'

The World Psychiatric Association Section on Spirituality and Religion in Psychiatry has since approved a landmark position statement on spirituality and religion in psychiatry.[4] Nevertheless, for the most part, the coming of age of psychiatry tells a story of unrelenting preoccupation with the neurobiology of mental illness to the exclusion of spiritual beliefs and values, and of heavy reliance on psychotropic medication in consort with the pharmaceutical industry.

It is hardly surprising, therefore, that mental health science is dismissive of indigenous peoples' understanding of spiritual reality as 'primitive' and 'animistic'. For instance, the shamanic view of 'spirit', which has informed cultures as far apart as Northern Asian and Mongolian tribes, the Inuit, North American Indians, the tribes of the Amazon Basin, the Aborigines of Australia and in Europe, the Celts, is these days of little interest other than to medical anthropologists.

Contemporary psychiatry treats the major faith traditions of today with much the same disregard. This becomes more intelligible in the light of Gallup surveys, which show that while around 80% of the general population believe in God or a 'force' or 'spirit',[5] only some 25% of psychiatrists do.[6] I shall be looking at some of the consequences for mental healthcare of this striking difference of view.

Spirituality in Western Antiquity

Every culture has a tendency to regard its achievements as pre-eminent and Western science is no exception. The real world is considered to

---

3. World Health Organization (1998: 7–8).
4. Moreira-Almeida et al. (2016).
5. Eurobarometer Poll (2005).
6. Neeleman & King (1993).

be the one that we can touch, feel, see, hear and taste, while metaphysical or supramundane reality is treated as mere imagination. Yet this fashionable belief system is just a few hundred years old, and derives entirely from instruments which themselves are composed of the same materials that they measure. It follows, naturally, that only matters of physical substance could thereby ever be substantiated!

Taking the part for the whole is a serious mistake. For this reason I want to situate the secularism of Western science within the broad sweep of other civilisations, which have nonetheless advanced their own traditions of scholarship, wisdom and truth. I shall use the word 'soul' to mean the unique and irreducible essence of each person, while by 'spirit' I will refer to the more general animating principle behind all of matter.[7]

The Greeks saw science and soul as going hand in hand. Pythagoras, born in the 6th century BCE, recalled an earlier incarnation as Euphorbus, a warrior in the Trojan War. In the 3rd century BCE, Socrates likewise asserted the immortality of the soul. His pupil Plato claimed that through virtuous living, the soul is purified and regains its original perfection, while moral dereliction leads to Tartarus (Hell). As to the true nature of reality, in his famous allegory of the cave, Plato likened our perception of reality to mistaking the shadows dancing on the cave wall for the puppets that cast the shadow.

Jewish mysticism (Kabbalah) also has a long and ancient history. 'Hidden teachings' were revealed by angels to Adam and handed down to Noah and Moses. According to the Zohar, souls must reincarnate until the germ planted in them grows to perfection, when they return to the Absolute. Islam, too, has its mystical tradition in Sufism, in which the 'rational' soul is regarded as eternal.

Eastern Metaphysics

Turning eastwards, we find the same belief in a transpersonal soul in Hinduism, rooted in the Vedas that go back 3500 years. The soul (*atman*) is caught in the cycle of birth and death until purification through yoga. Only then, free from *sanskars* (past impressions), will the soul finally attain union with Brahman, the Divine Ground of existence.

---

7. It appears that earlier civilisations have always believed in the existence of animating life energy: the Egyptians called it *ka*, the Greeks *psyche* and the Romans *spiritus*.

Taoism,[8] which was refined in the 6th century BCE in China, teaches of the *Tao*, often translated as 'The Way', a path of perfect balance, in harmony with cosmic law and represented by the *Taiji*, the symbol of *yin* and *yang* entwined together. The soul is understood to be composed of two parts, *kwei*, which is terrestrial and impermanent, and *shen*, celestial and immortal.

The third great Eastern spiritual tradition is Buddhism, originating in India in the 5th century BCE and spreading to China 200 years later. Central to the Buddha's teachings is overcoming the inevitable suffering that life brings through reaching the state of *annata* ('no-self'), liberating the mundane self from karma (the burdensome consequences of the law of cause and effect). Buddhists hold that nothing of the (illusory) ego or self has permanence, so there can be no continuity of the individual soul beyond death. Rebirth is essentially impersonal, and since Buddhists see preoccupation with individual survival beyond death as a function of the ego (from which further suffering must arise), speculation about an afterlife is not encouraged.[9]

Christian Religion: Dogma or Revelation?

Early Gnostic texts, such as the gospels of Thomas and Philip and the Pistis Sophia, all refer to reincarnation. However, the four synoptic gospels of Matthew, Mark, Luke and John offer no more than hints. The first blow against reincarnation was dealt by the Roman emperor Constantine at the Council of Nicea in 325, when Jesus Christ was declared the *only* son of God according to the Nicene Creed. At a stroke, the human race was set apart and subordinated to the Church, requiring the priest to intercede for the sins of humanity. In 543, at the 5th General Council of Churches convened by the Emperor Justinian, the doctrine of reincarnation was explicitly condemned, probably because the notion of rebirth challenged the hierarchy of Roman power and privilege. Gnosis (direct revelation of the Divine) also came to be seen as potentially subversive. Instead, strict adherence to the approved teachings of the Church was given prominence.

Following the fall of the Roman Empire, mediaeval Europe was dominated by Roman Catholicism, unified until 1054, when the Great

---

8. Also known as Daoism.
9. The exception is Tibetan Buddhism, which has a detailed iconography of the after-death world or *bardo*, an intermediate realm prior to rebirth. See Evans-Wentz (1960).

Schism took place that divided the Roman Catholic and Eastern Orthodox Churches. Shortly after, Pope Urban II started the first crusade in defence of the Christian Byzantine Empire, which was under attack by Muslim Seljuk Turks. A century of war followed, foreshadowing Christian intolerance of both heresy and the religions of Judaism and Islam, leading in 1478 to the Spanish Inquisition, which was not rescinded until 1834.

Despite the institutional politics of a church that demanded conformity and absolute obedience, the mystical tradition has nevertheless been upheld by individuals who trusted their own relationship with God more than fealty to the established order. The list includes Hildegard of Bingen, Francis of Assisi, Meister Eckhart, Julian of Norwich, Martin Luther, St. John of the Cross, Jakob Boehme, Blaise Pascal, Emanuel Swedenborg, Pierre Teilhard de Chardin and Thomas Merton. Psychiatrists should be aware of this revelatory mystical tradition, for their patients are less likely to bring the catechism to the consulting room than personal revelations of God and sometimes the devil too. Indeed, in an increasingly multi-ethnic society, psychiatrists need to be conversant with all the major faith traditions.[10]

The Scourge of Evil and the Fate of the Mentally Ill

In the Middle Ages, the prospect was not good for those suffering from serious mental disorder. In England, the first Act of Parliament against witchcraft was passed in 1401. The water test was used: the accused were bound hand and foot and thrown into a pond. Those who sank (and usually drowned) were declared innocent, while those who floated were found guilty and burned at the stake.

A further Act of Parliament followed in 1604, which determined 'death without benefit of clergy to anyone who invoked evil spirits or communed with familiar spirits'. Around 1000 people, mostly women, were put to death in England and Wales (some 40,000 in all of Europe) prior to the 1735 Witchcraft Act of George III, when hanging was replaced with imprisonment. The Act was not repealed until 1951, seven years after it was last used to prosecute the medium Helen Duncan, found guilty and imprisoned for nine months for allegedly betraying details of the D-Day preparations via 'pretended' contacts with the spirit world.

---

10. Salem & Foskett (2009).

The Renaissance

At the turn of the 15th century, Copernicus was the first to challenge the geocentric world-view of Catholicism. A century later, Galileo Galilei was sentenced to house arrest for daring to assert, with the aid of his telescope, that the planets of the solar system moved around the sun. The force for change, however, was inexorable, and before long the doctrinal cosmology of the Church was broken.

René Descartes claimed that nothing can be held to be true until one is absolutely certain of it. Since the one thing Descartes could not doubt was his own existence, he gave primacy of mind over matter: *cogito, ergo sum*. Yet Descartes also said that to be capable of so perfect an idea as God meant that such an idea could not have been caused by anything less perfect than God! Isaac Newton, who described the laws of gravitation and motion in his great work *Principia Mathematica*, was also deeply religious, holding the universe to be the work of God.

The profound discoveries of Descartes and Newton set in motion a revolution that by the 18th century led to the Age of Enlightenment, with a flowering of individualism in the arts, in political and social reform, and with extraordinary progress in science, medicine and technology. At the same time, fateful seeds had been sown, for Descartes' dictum, ill-used, served to put Man in place of God and Newton's physics were employed to relegate God to a Heaven that had no substance except in faith. The result was the birth of material realism, which since that time has taken humankind down a path of alienation from both the spiritual universe and the wisdom of Nature. Here are some of the consequences that we live with today.

- Empirical science does not give weight to subjective experience. The only reality is the world 'out there', which can be objectively appraised. Events take place by chance and only become statistically meaningful when they can be shown to have significantly deviated from chance occurrence.
- Since science is reductive/analytic, a concept such as 'wholeness' has little heuristic value.
- Causation is 'bottom up' rather than 'top down'; it follows that consciousness must somehow be generated by the activity of brain cells (although, as yet, no one knows how).
- The value of altered states of consciousness, requiring a different research methodology, is discounted in favour of a uniform 'consensus reality'.

- Despite advances in quantum physics, which show all 'reality' to be subjective, the ideal of objectivity remains the touchstone of science (the 'Newtonian' world-view).

In just a few hundred years, Western civilisation has traded the subjective, intuitive and sacred for the objective, rational and secular – the epic myth of our time.[11] Yet the prevalence of mental illness, far from abating, is increasing.

Pioneers of Humanitarian Care for the Mentally Ill

Until the 18th century, people living in Europe who were considered 'mad' (but not deemed to be witches or possessed by the devil) were incarcerated. The Bethlem Royal Hospital, where inmates were put in chains and publicly ridiculed, had been founded in Britain as early as 1247 and was popularly known as Bedlam.

A small number of influential reformers finally prevailed over this inhuman treatment. In Paris, Phillipe Pinel instigated 'moral treatment', first at Bicêtre Hospital and then at the Hospice de la Salpêtrière. Pinel stopped the use of purging, blistering and bleeding, preferring to talk with his patients. Independently, in England, William Tuke, a Quaker, founded The Retreat in York, caring for the afflicted with humanity and concern. John Conolly, who became the superintendent of Hanwell Asylum in the suburbs of London, published a ground-breaking book in 1856 entitled *Treatment of the Insane without Mechanical Restraints*, advocated providing patients with both occupational and recreational activities, and insisted they should be treated with kindness.[12]

Care of the Mentally Ill in the 19th Century

By the 19th century, mental illness had come to be seen as a medical problem and the treatment given was, for the most part, humane. However, an experiment in social engineering had been taking place through the building of parliament-funded mental asylums, which

---

11. Philosopher and scientist Bernadino Kastrup writes: 'Myth is the code that each one of us constantly uses, whether we are aware of it or not, to interpret life in the world [...] To say that nature is a mechanical apparatus without purpose or intentionality is itself an interpretation; a myth' (2016: 18–19).
12. Conolly (1856).

segregated and isolated the patient population. By 1930, over 140,000 patients were living in such institutions in the UK.

Some patients benefited; those too disturbed to care for themselves could become part of a community, working on the hospital estate and taking part in the asylum's organised recreational life. Many others suffered greatly, having been inappropriately diagnosed in the first place or confined for spurious social reasons, including the diagnosis of 'moral degeneracy', or simply because they had nowhere else to go. Shamefully, large numbers of patients were effectively subjected to a lifetime's confinement with no means of appeal.

Psychiatry in the 20th Century

By the end of the 19th century, a range of physical causes had been shown to be responsible for mental disorder, including infections (e.g. neurosyphilis), anatomical lesions (tumours and head injuries), biochemical disorders (e.g. porphyria) and vitamin deficiencies (thiamine and B12). The classification of severe mental illness into two types, schizophrenia and manic depression (bipolar disorder), encouraged psychiatrists to believe that the underlying causes would soon be found.[13]

Early 20th-century treatments included medication with opiates, bromides and barbiturates. However, from the 1940s and over the next two decades, lobotomy, a procedure that could be carried out in ten minutes in a doctor's consulting room, was widely performed (40,000 in the USA, 17,000 in the UK).[14] Insulin coma therapy was also popular, another intervention that destroyed brain tissue, this time with glucose and oxygen starvation. Both treatments wrecked many thousands of lives.

Electroconvulsive therapy (ECT), discovered in 1938, soon became a mainstay of treatment. Around 12,000 treatments per year

---

13. Today, the case for schizophrenia being a single disease entity is losing ground. The neuropathology may represent a common final pathway resulting from the impact of multiple stressors, both physical and emotional. See Murray (2017). Neither is bipolar disorder proving to be a single disease entity – for a summary of bipolar sub-types, see Chernick (2017).
14. 'Ice-pick' lobotomies were invented by Dr Walter Freeman, who toured the USA in his self-styled 'lobotomobile'. The patient was first rendered unconscious by an electroconvulsive shock, then a probe was angled upwards in each eye socket and hammered through the skull into the frontal cortex of the brain. Many patients were left with permanent brain damage and the mortality rate was around 15%.

are still given in the UK on the grounds that ECT can relieve intractable depression where medication has failed and when, for example, the patient is severely agitated, delusional, suicidal, not eating or drinking, or suffering from life-threatening catatonia. There continues to be a vociferous critique against ECT, alleging its unethical and inappropriate use.[15]

From the 1950s onwards, an ever increasing pharmacopeia has been available for the treatment of mental disorders.[16] Antipsychotic drugs became available for schizophrenia, tricyclic antidepressants came on the market, benzodiazepines were widely used for the treatment of anxiety, and the mood stabiliser lithium was given for manic depression, as it was then called. In the 1960s, a new class of antidepressants, the monoamine oxidase inhibitors (MAOIs), was discovered and since then two further classes of antidepressants have been marketed: the selective serotonin reuptake inhibitors (SSRIs) and the serotonin and norepinephrine reuptake inhibitors (SNRIs), as well as numerous second and third generation antipsychotics.[17]

Evaluating the effectiveness of this therapeutic armamentarium has been complex. Benefits have to be weighed against often serious side-effects; the therapeutic response is highly individual and even then must be distinguished from the placebo effect. Not least, we live in a culture where medication is frequently turned to as a catch-all for unhappiness.[18] While psychiatric medication never cures, symptoms may be alleviated, giving time for natural recovery when possible. There is now evidence that short-term drug treatments can provide moderate benefit in cases of severe mental illness, but that long-term use of both antidepressants[19] and antipsychotics[20,21] may worsen outcome.

In parallel with early physical methods of treatment, psychoanalysis had been *the* psychological therapy of the first half of the century. However, from the 1960s onwards, psychoanalysis lost out, on the one hand to pharmacotherapy and on the other hand to behaviour therapy (later to become cognitive–behavioural therapy or CBT).[22]

---

15. Johnstone (2003).
16. There has, of course, been a comparable burgeoning of medical pharmaceuticals as a whole.
17. For a powerful critique of the pharmaceutical approach to mental illness, see Davies (2013).
18. See *Recovery and Well-Being: The Search for the Soul*, this volume.
19. For a concise summary, see Kaplan (2012).
20. Insel (2013).
21. Wunderink et al. (2013).
22. Hofmann et al. (2012).

On the matter of religion, biological psychiatry, psychoanalysis and behavioural therapy were all of a like mind: none had any time for it.[23] Nevertheless, towards the end of the 20th century, there was a revival of interest in the relationship between spirituality and mental health. Of note was a large body of research emanating from the USA and demonstrating a positive correlation between spirituality, religion and mental health.[24] Further, user-led mental health charities in the UK were asking for spiritual aspects of care to be valued,[25] including recognition of the 'spiritual emergency'.[26] In the wider cultural milieu, too, there was new interest in the health benefits of meditation.[27] Not least, there was a resurgence of interest in transpersonal psychology and this is what I want to focus upon here.

As a psychological therapy, the transpersonal approach has its origins in the analytical psychology of Carl Jung, while also drawing on the great religious and mystical traditions for spiritual illumination. However, in the UK, analytical psychology has influenced mental healthcare to only a small extent, there being so few Jungian-trained consultants in the National Health Service (NHS). Further, the Jungian approach is traditionally less concerned with symptom resolution than with 'individuation', the development of the 'whole person'. Such in-depth exploration not only of personality but also of the deeper self or soul is out of step with the short-term treatments approved and funded by the NHS.

Soul-centred approaches can, nevertheless, be integrated into clinical practice, as I describe elsewhere.[28] Moreover, the willingness of the patient to work transpersonally may be readily elicited by taking a spiritual history – a subject to which I shall be returning.

In summary, the main influences on contemporary psychiatry can be outlined as follows:

---

23. A leading psychiatric textbook used for three decades contains just two references to religion, 'religiosity in deteriorated epileptic' and 'religious belief, neurotic search for'. See Mayer-Gross et al. (1955).
24. Koenig et al. (2001).
25. Faulkner (1997).
26. A term coined by Stanislav Grof (Grof & Grof, 1989).
27. Later formalised as mindfulness-meditation. See Kabat-Zinn (1996).
28. See *Soul-Centred Psychotherapy*, this volume.

| Biological Psychiatry | Psychoanalysis (Freud) | Analytical Psychology (Jung) |

Biological psychiatry and psychoanalysis in rivalry but both prejudiced against spirituality and religion

Perls, Moreno, Assagioli, Grof, Wilber

Psychology CBT

Shamanic Mystical and Established Faith Traditions Spiritism, Near Death Experience Research

Physical/pharmaceutical treatments

Mindfulness based therapy
Psychotherapy

Transpersonal Therapies
Spirit Release, Soul Retrieval, Psychosynthesis, Holotropic Breathwork, Past Life and Between Lives, Therapies, Soul-centred Psychotherapy

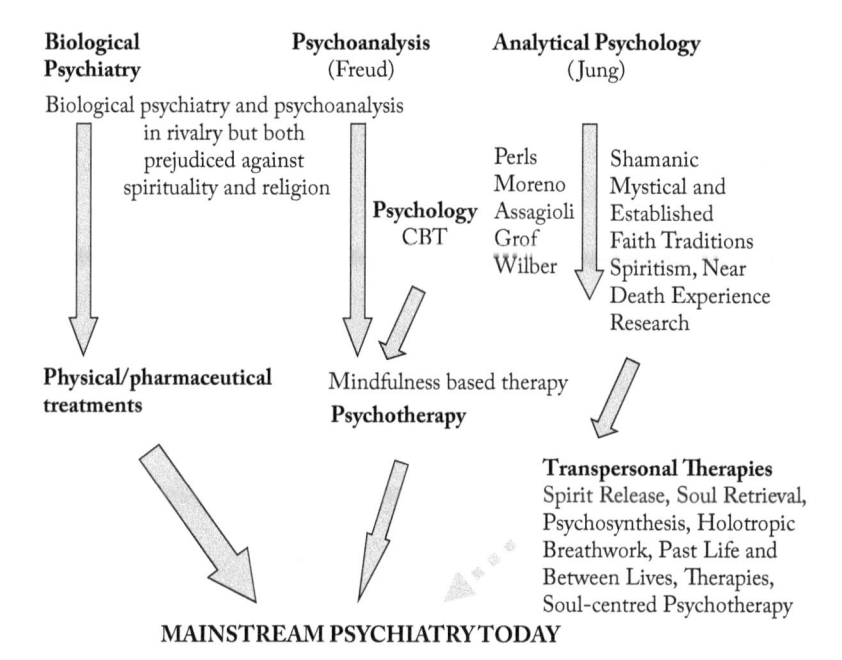

MAINSTREAM PSYCHIATRY TODAY

4.1. Mainstream psychiatry. Arrow size illustrates influences on current practice.

Mental Illness – A Crisis of Modernity

Mental disorder in the UK has now assumed epidemic proportions. Surveys in England have shown that one in four adults experience a mental health problem each year,[29] with one in six in any given week experiencing a common mental health problem (such as anxiety and depression).[30] In England and Wales, one in eight adults receives treatment for a mental health problem.[31]

What is going wrong? Is the human race suffering from some kind of biological meltdown? Is it just that the burgeoning classification of mental disorders means there is more 'pathology' to be diagnosed? Or could it be that modernity, with its incessant materialistic and secular pursuits, is estranging people from their spiritual core and the innate values of truth, beauty and goodness?[32] If so, small wonder that the stage is set for breakdown, whether the health of the individual,

---

29. McManus et al. (2009).
30. McManus et al. (2016).
31. See Welsh Government (2016).
32. Derived from Platonic idealism, a triad known as the 'transcendentals'.

society or indeed the ecology of the planet – all symptoms of a profound spiritual crisis.

Stanislav Grof, who founded the Spiritual Emergency Network at the Esalen Institute in 1980, summarises thus:

> '...there exist spontaneous non-ordinary states of consciousness (NOSC) that would in the West be seen and treated as psychosis, and treated mostly by suppressive medication. But if we use the observations from the study of non-ordinary states, and also from other spiritual traditions, they should really be treated as crises of transformation, or crises of spiritual opening. Something that should really be supported rather than suppressed. If properly understood and properly supported, they are actually conducive to healing and transformation'.[33]

Spiritual emergencies can present to the psychiatrist in a variety of ways, and not necessarily with psychosis.[34] It is easiest to help those patients who can recognise how their symptoms relate to loss of meaning and purpose in life and who welcome a spiritually informed therapeutic approach.

A second group presents with a range of emotional or somatic symptoms of spiritual origin, which include Kundalini.[35] Here, it is important that the psychiatrist does not prematurely diagnose mental illness, which can happen if the spiritual practices of the patient have not been taken into account.

Many psychiatrists would argue that there is an overlap between the spiritual emergency and schizophrenia of acute onset. When a patient presents with psychotic symptoms that have strong religious or spiritual significance, the evaluation can be problematic. There is no diagnostic entry in the World Health Organization's *International Classification of Diseases* (ICD-10) for 'spiritual emergency'.[36] There is, however, an entry for acute and transient psychotic disorders (ATPD; F23), described as follows:

> 'A heterogeneous group of disorders characterized by the acute onset of psychotic symptoms such as delusions, hallucinations, and perceptual disturbances, and by the severe disruption of ordinary behaviour. Acute

---

33. Redwood (1995).
34. Crowley (2005).
35. First referred to in early Hindu texts, Kundalini is experienced as an uncontrollable surge of energy accompanied by involuntary motor and sensory reactions and often in an altered state of consciousness. When sought through meditation, the aim is awakening to bliss. However, Kundalini can arise spontaneously, and in the unstable and vulnerable individual can lead to psychosis. See *Varieties of Love and the Near-Life Experience*, in Powell (2017); also Sanella (1987).
36. For a full discussion of this diagnostic issue, see Teodorescu (2009).

onset is defined as a crescendo development of a clearly abnormal clinical picture in about two weeks or less ... Complete recovery usually occurs within a few months, often within a few weeks or even days. If the disorder persists, a change in classification will be necessary. The disorder may or may not be associated with acute stress, defined as usually stressful events preceding the onset by one to two weeks'.[37]

People suffering from ATPD recover, by definition, from the episode of illness. However, there is a significant relapse rate and one in eight individuals with first-ever diagnosed ATPD will develop schizophrenia within 3-5 years.[38]

Because most psychiatrists are not attuned to the spiritual dimension, we do not know how many of such patients are breaking down because of a spiritual crisis, and neither do we know to what extent an informed psycho-spiritual intervention might engender a good outcome. One problem in particular is that intense spiritual preoccupations are often treated by the psychiatrist as a feature of illness and therefore to be discouraged. Nevertheless, the embattled archetypes of good and evil that so often figure in the time of crisis do need to be addressed, for if the inner struggle is left to continue unaided, it generally erupts again. The skill lies in finding a creative way to help the patient work with his/her spiritual concerns that may protect against further breakdown.[39]

Furthering Spirituality in Psychiatry in the UK

Over the years, and as my interest in the psychology of spirituality deepened, I increasingly felt something must be done to promote the need for more spiritually informed mental healthcare. With clinical training and practice being so geared to the secular world-view, there seemed little consideration of the spiritual dimension other than a tick-box approach to religion. Talking to colleagues revealed that a good many were unhappy with the limitations imposed by the prevailing dogma of scientific realism. Neither was there a professional forum in which seriously to question such matters without risking censure.

Surveys had showed that over one half of patients turn to their spirituality/religion to help them at times of crisis. Further, archetypal spiritual/religious themes often feature in mental illness. It seemed to me that for a well-informed and accurate diagnosis to be made, the

---

37. World Health Organization (2010).
38. Queirazza et al. (2014).
39. For a lively account of work in this field, see Clarke (2008). See also the Spiritual Crisis Network (http://spiritualcrisisnetwork.uk).

psychiatrist needs to be able to explore this hinterland in such a way as to gain and deserve the trust of the patient. This is all the harder to do if the psychiatrist knows nothing about the faith tradition of the patient. Moreover, if the psychiatrist is unaware of research that shows the benefit of spirituality and religion to mental health, the whole subject is more than likely to be glossed over.

I concluded that the best way forward was to form an interest group in spirituality and psychiatry, one that would align psychiatry with its intended meaning of *psyche* (soul) and *iatros* (doctor). Sympathetic colleagues were canvassed and a proposal was put to the Royal College of Psychiatrists, where happily it found support. In 1999, the Spirituality and Psychiatry Special Interest Group (SPSIG) held its inaugural meeting and convened its first conference in January 2000. Since then, the membership has grown apace.[40]

From the start, the SPSIG has aimed to provide a discussion forum for psychiatrists to explore a wide range of subjects, including existential questions about the purpose and meaning of life, the problem of good and evil, near-death, mystical and trance states, paranormal phenomena, the 'spiritual emergency', differences between healthy and unhealthy spirituality, and the evidence base for spirituality and religion improving mental health outcomes.

There are wider implications too, such as the effects of meditation, prayer and altered states of consciousness; the spiritual significance of anxiety, doubt, guilt and shame on the one hand and love, altruism and forgiveness on the other; and how the prevailing culture of consumerism and materialism affects personal identity and self-esteem.

The SPSIG has consistently advocated taking a spiritual history as part of the clinical assessment,[41] enabling the psychiatrist to find out whether the patient's spirituality or religion is felt as supportive or stressful, how it affects the way the person sees their problem, if there are spiritual or religious issues the patient would like to discuss in therapy and when support from chaplaincy would be helpful.[42]

In order to inform as widely as possible, the SPSIG website is entirely in the public domain, a newsletter is published regularly, there are conferences twice yearly and the website archive holds over 200 papers written by psychiatrists that can be freely downloaded. Two

---

40. The membership in 2017 stands at more than 3000 psychiatrists. See http://www.rcpsych.ac.uk/spirit
41. See Eagger (2011).
42. The value of the spiritual assessment was recognised by the College with the publication of *Recommendations for Psychiatrists on Spirituality and Religion* (Royal College of Psychiatrists, 2013).

books have subsequently been published on the subject of spirituality and mental health by the College.[43]

As to the future, among other things is the need to highlight current research on the non-local nature of consciousness that offers a new understanding of anomalous perceptual experiences. More research is needed into the efficacy of a range of psycho-spiritual approaches, including soul centred therapies, together with opportunity for appropriate training.[44]

The broad approach of the SPSIG has always been holistic. Medical intervention in the case of serious mental disorder can be lifesaving. Nevertheless, for the deepest healing to take place, we need to engage the soul, as happens when we gently enquire into a person's spiritual values and beliefs.

Psychiatry, as with all of medicine, should be guided by the golden rule: 'Do to others as you would have them do to you'.[45] Doctor and patient are in complementary roles – each needs the other. We are all travelling down the path of learning, one that ultimately takes us to the same destination. Furthermore, we can remain optimistic in the most apparently hopeless cases, for in the bigger picture we cannot know what the outcome must be – only that we do our best to help. Not least, and always at our disposal, is the best medicine known to humankind – the healing power of love.

References

Chernick, D. (2007) A snapshot of bipolar depression subtypes. Available at: https://www.medpagetoday.com/resource-center/bipolar-resource-center/bipolar-depression-subtypes/a/63892 (accessed 4 July 2017).

Clarke, I. (2008) *Madness, Mystery and the Survival of God*. O Books.

Conolly, J. (1856) *The Treatment Of The Insane Without Mechanical Restraints*. Reprinted [2013]. Cambridge University Press.

Cook, C.C.H., Powell, A. & Sims, A. (2009) *Spirituality and Psychiatry*. RCPsych Publications.

Cook, C.C.H., Powell, A. & Sims, A. (2016) *Spirituality and Narrative in Psychiatric Practice*. RCPsych Publications.

Crowley, N. (2005) Psychosis or spiritual emergence? Consideration of the transpersonal perspective within psychiatry. Available at: http://www.rcpsych.ac.uk/spsigarchive

---

43. Cook et al. (2009; 2016).
44. Mindfulness-based cognitive therapy has now become recognised as an approved treatment for anxiety and the prevention of relapse of depression. See Williams & Kabat-Zinn (2013).
45. Luke 6:31. *The Holy Bible*, NIV.

Davies, J. (2013) *Cracked: Why Psychiatry is Doing More Harm Than Good.* Icon Books.
Eagger, S. (2011) Spirituality in psychiatry: implementing spiritual assessment. Available at: http://www.rcpsych.ac.uk/spsigarchive
Eurobarometer Poll (2005) Bar chart for beliefs. Available at: https://commons.wikimedia.org/wiki/File:Eurobarometer_poll.png (accessed 4 July 2017).
Evans-Wentz, W.Y. (1960) *The Tibetan Book of the Dead.* Oxford University Press.
Faulkner, A. (1997) *Knowing Our Own Minds.* Mental Health Foundation.
Grof, S. & Grof, C. (1989) *Spiritual Emergency: When Personal Transformation Becomes A Crisis.* Tarcher.
Hofmann, S., Asnaani, A., Imke, M., et al. (2012) The efficacy of cognitive behavioral therapy: a review of meta-analyses. *Cognitive Therapy and Research*, 36, 427–440.
Insel, T. (2013) Antipsychotics: taking the long view [blog]. Available at: https://www.nimh.nih.gov/about/directors/thomas-insel/blog/2013/antipsychotics-taking-the-long-view.shtml (accessed 4 July 2017).
Johnstone, L. (2003) A shocking treatment. *The Psychologist*, 16, 236-239.
Kabat-Zinn, J. (1996) *Full Catastrophe Living: How to Cope with Stress, Pain and Illness Using Mindfulness Meditation.* Piatkus.
Kaplan, A. (2012) On the efficacy of psychiatric drugs. *Psychiatric Times*, 3 April. Available at: http://www.psychiatrictimes.com/articles/efficacy-psychiatric-drugs (accessed 4 July 2017).
Kastrup, B. (2016) *More than Allegory: On Religious Myth, Truth and Belief.* iff Books.
Koenig, H.K., McCullough, M.E. & Larson, D.B. (2001) *Handbook of Religion and Health.* Oxford University Press.
Mayer-Gross, W., Slater, E. & Roth, M. (1955) *Clinical Psychiatry.* Cassell.
McManus, S., Meltzer, H., Brugha, T.S., et al. (2009) *Adult Psychiatric Morbidity in England, 2007: Results of a Household Survey.* NHS Health and Social Care Information Centre.
McManus, S., Bebbington, P., Jenkins, R., et al. (eds) (2016) *Mental Health and Wellbeing in England: Adult Psychiatric Morbidity Survey 2014.* NHS Digital.
Moreira-Almeida, A., Sharma, A., van Rensburg, B.J., et al. (2016) WPA position statement on spirituality and religion in psychiatry. *World Psychiatry*, 15, 87–88.
Murray, R. (2017) Mistakes I have made in my research career. *Schizophrenia Bulletin*, 43, 253–256.
Neeleman, J. & King, M.B. (1993) Psychiatrists' religious attitudes in relation to their clinical practice: a survey of 231 psychiatrists. *Acta Psychiatrica Scandinavica*, 88, 420–424.
Powell, A. (2017) *The Ways of the Soul. A Psychiatrist Reflects: Essays on Life, Death and Beyond.* Muswell Hill Press.
Queirazza, F., Semple, D., Semple, M., et al. (2014) Transition to schizophrenia in acute and transient psychotic disorders. *British Journal of Psychiatry*, 204(4), 299-305.
Redwood, D. (1995) Frontiers of the Mind: Interview with Stanislav Grof MD. Healthy.net. Available at: http://www.healthy.net/scr/interview.aspx?Id=200 (accessed 4 July 2017).
Royal College of Psychiatrists (2013) *Recommendations for Psychiatrists on Spirituality and Religion* (Position Statement PS03/2013). RCPsych.
Salem, M. & Foskett, J. (2009) Religion and religious experiences. In *Spirituality and Psychiatry* (eds C.C.H. Cook, A. Powell & A. Sims). RCPsych Publications.
Sanella, L. (1987) *The Kundalini Experience: Transcendence or Psychosis.* Integral Publishing.

Teodorescu, D. (2009) ICD-10's limitations to distinguish between psychosis and spiritual emergencies: the need for a new diagnosis in ICD-11 for spiritual or religious problems. Available at: https://www.scribd.com/document/59145254/ICD-11article-by-Dinu-Teodorescu-2009 (accessed 4 July 2017).

Welsh Government (2016) Welsh Health Survey 2015: Health Status, Illnesses, and Other Conditions. *Statistical Bulletin*, 24, 1–40. Available at: http://gov.wales/docs/statistics/2016/160622-welsh-health-survey-2015-health-status-illnesses-other-conditions-en.pdf (accessed 18 September 2017).

Williams, M. & Kabat-Zinn, J. (2013) *Mindfulness*. Routledge.

World Health Organization (1998) *WHOQOL and Spirituality, Religiousness and Personal Beliefs (SRPB)*. WHO. Available at: http://apps.who.int/iris/bitstream/10665/70897/1/WHO_MSA_MHP_98.2_eng.pdf (accessed 4 July 2017).

World Health Organization (2010) *International Statistical Classification of Diseases and Related Health Problems, 10th Revision* (ICD-10). WHO.

Wunderink, L., Nieboer, R., Wiersma, D., et al. (2013) Recovery in remitted first-episode psychosis at 7 years of follow-up of an early dose reduction/discontinuation or maintenance treatment strategy: long-term follow-up of a 2-year randomized clinical trial. *JAMA Psychiatry*, 70(9), 913–920.

5

Past Life Memory – A Key to Understanding the Self?

When asked to speak about 'past lives' at a conference on 'Self and Death – What Survives?' my first thought was simply to give an account of the therapy popularly known as past life regression. Then I realised that to do justice to the subject, I would need to say something about the worldly or mundane, egoic self, its relation to the spiritual self or soul, and how past life regression is able to help the mundane self to see its life story through the eyes of the soul. To set the scene, however, I will begin with a short past life memory of my own:

> With the other men of my tribe, I am standing on the earthwork rampart that encircles our village. The women and children are hiding inside the dwellings. We are armed with spears and clubs, waiting for the attack that is coming. Suddenly, with terrible shouting, it is upon us, fierce and brutal. Many are killed on both sides – no mercy is expected or shown. Then it is over, as quickly as it started and we men return to our huts, completely exhausted. My woman tenderly rubs herbs on my wounds and I lie down on a bed of heather. I know that the next day there will be more fighting but tonight we are safe.
>
> At dawn the attack starts up again. We are outnumbered but fight to the end. I feel a spear go into my back and know I am dying. As I lie unable to move, I see the marauders swarm into the enclosure, raping and killing our women and children. My physical pain is nothing compared with the pain of seeing the brutal murder of my kith and kin, and my failure to protect them. As death comes, I find myself floating up, leaving my body where it lies. Then I am astonished to see, rising upwards from all over the enclosure, the souls of everyone, young and old, who have been massacred. Their bodies remain where they have

Paper prepared for conference 'Beyond the Brain VIII: Self and Death – What Survives?' held by the Scientific and Medical Network in association with the Spirituality and Psychiatry Special Interest Group, Royal College of Psychiatrists, Canterbury, August 2009.

fallen but together they are ascending, apparently unharmed, into the light. Joining them, I leave this terrible scene of death.

The enduring impression made on me by this past life memory – one of the first I experienced – was not the massacre itself but the sight of souls leaving the scene of carnage, and my leaving with them. I will say more about the importance of going 'beyond death' in the examples of past lives I shall give later.

In drawing a conceptual map, albeit a rather simple one, I will look first at how the mundane self is established, then at its relationship with the spiritual self, briefly consider what kinds of conscious reality may exist beyond death and conclude with three short accounts of past lives of my own. I hope to illustrate how the ego can thereby find a greater understanding of life and the challenges that come its way.

Acquiring a Self

From the start of life, the human mind has an extraordinary propensity to search for meaning, thereby assembling a picture of the world that brings order to what otherwise would be an overwhelming kaleidoscope of sensory impressions.[1] We cannot really know what it is like to be a baby. Reconstruction through re-birthing, primal therapy and hypnotic regression takes us close, but the infant processes data differently from the adult and observational studies of child development can only show us the surface of things rather than the inward experience. Nevertheless, many would concur that there is a preternatural wisdom to be seen in the eyes of a newborn infant.[2] To paraphrase William Blake, the baby appears to see not *with* but *through* the eye.[3] The soul of the infant is visible, naked, wondering and curious about the strange world it has entered.

To begin with, a baby is unaware of the difference between inside and outside, self and other. Gradually, the baby learns to differentiate, as when it puts a finger in its mother's mouth and then its own, comparing the difference in sensation. Over time a body schema develops

---

1. The writings of Franz Kafka chillingly portray the threat to the self when a person is unable to make sense of what is going on. Delusion formation due to severe mental illness can be understood as a desperate attempt to reclaim some kind of coherent identity when ego boundaries have become permeable to chaotic and often frightening sensory impressions.
2. For further discussion, see *The Soul of the Newborn Child*, in Powell (2017).
3. Blake (1917: 175).

that is confirmed when the child discovers its own reflection in a mirror and sees itself delimited by the boundary of its own skin.

The child's mind is not similarly confined, for it learns to reach into the minds of others, becoming aware of their beliefs and intentions. Theory of Mind suggests that we are hard-wired to exercise this astonishing ability of sensing another's world.[4] At the same time, the healthy child remains centred in its growing sense of individuality.

This is most likely why toddlers learn to say 'no' before they say 'yes'. There are deep implications for the privacy of the self. No one person's truth can belong to anyone else, since 'reality' can only be apprehended subjectively. However, it helps for one person's reality to be at least comprehensible to others. When personal reality diverges too far from consensus reality, especially where there is suffering, mental disorder is not infrequently diagnosed.

Past, Present and Future

Children live largely in the 'now', something that many grown-ups, constantly distracted with tasks and duties, wish they could discover anew. Omar Khayyám, the 11th-century Persian poet, mathematician and philosopher, chides us:[5]

> 'Oh, come with old Khayyám, and leave the Wise
> To talk: one thing is certain, that Life flies;
> One thing is certain, and the rest is Lies;
> The Flower that once has blown for ever dies.
>
> [and]
>
> Ah, fill the Cup: – what boots it to repeat
> How Time is slipping underneath our Feet:
> Unborn TO-MORROW, and dead YESTERDAY,
> Why fret about them if TO-DAY be sweet!'

Fully to embrace the 'now' is an act that is unconditional and unconditioned. Furthermore, the 'now', of itself, does not exist within time,[6]

---

4. Except, that is, for children with autistic spectrum disorder, who are unable to develop the capacity for empathic identification with others and consequently remain profoundly self-referenced. For more on Theory of Mind, see Baron-Cohen et al. (1999).
5. Fitzgerald (1989).
6. As experienced, for instance, in *samadhi* (Hinduism and Buddhism) or *satori* (Zen), in which the realisation of the 'now' is unbounded by space and time; a

and from this perspective, the past and the future exist only as mental constructs.

In ordinary waking consciousness these constructs are, of course, felt as entirely real. The moment my mind sets in motion the movement of thought, I become the protagonist of my life drama, in possession of a complex life story overflowing with all I have felt, thought, said and done. This is all in the possession of my ego,[7] which drives and directs my mundane self. Yet despite the ego's grand designs, the physical body from adulthood onwards is a constant reminder of entropy and decline. The arrow of time is relentless in its flight and seeks out beggars and kings alike – a powerful antidote to personal conceit. Omar Khayyám drives the point home:

> 'Think, in this batter'd Caravanserai
> Whose Doorways are alternate Night and Day,
> How Sultan after Sultan with his Pomp
> Abode his Hour or two and went his way.'

Precognition of death deeply alarms the ego, which fights it with an armoury of defence mechanisms. Sigmund Freud concluded that the death instinct, like an underground river sweeping us from birth to death, must necessarily be relegated to the unconscious. On the other hand, Carl Jung's view was entirely different. He saw the majestic archetype of the Self as transcending the limitations of the ego, fully able to accept and embrace life and death in turn.

From childhood onwards, the ego takes the lead in forging an individual's personality – the sum total of all traits, habits of mind and conditioning that shape a person's disposition. However, personality is not something fixed, for the mundane self is constantly in a web of relationships that feed and influence the experience of who a person takes themselves to be. Indeed, every human relationship draws from each person a unique response that is finely attuned to the other.

In this sense, the self can be compared to a musical ensemble. When musicians play well together, the music is greater than the sum of the parts – a harmony of wholeness arises. Not so, however, when the self becomes fragmented, as happens when traumatic events become split-off and lie dormant in the recesses of the psyche, sometimes for years, until they are triggered by a precipitating event. The problem for the wounded psyche is that as long as the trauma is left

---

state of pure awareness that precludes all thought, for thinking requires time (for the flow of thoughts) and space (through which the mind roams).

7. To this end, the ego is deeply attached to the possessive pronoun, hence: *my* body, *my* self, *my* life and *my* future.

unattended, a person cannot heal. Bearing this in mind, I want briefly to compare and contrast the mundane or egoic self with the spiritual self or soul.

The Mundane Self

As I earlier intimated, the ego is firmly rooted in the narrative of the past, from birth to the present day. Based on its history, the ego also invests heavily in the imagined future, affording a sense of direction, even a measure of control over what will happen next – something that gives it great comfort. While it is always possible I will be run over by a bus tomorrow, the egoic mind can find consolation in thinking that I would have had such and such a future, if only I hadn't been run over by the bus!

In this way, the ego functions in accordance with the laws of classical physics, situating itself in a physical world governed by events that follow one after another; a world of cause and effect. We can expect the sun to rise tomorrow, as it did today, yesterday and all the days before. More than that, such is the nature of the mundane self that we each experience ourselves to be at the epicentre of not only our own lives, but also of the whole world.

Yet there is poignancy about this Newtonian, egoic self, securely nested in space and time, for it relates to other selves like ships that pass in the night. The closest we can get to each other physically is when we make love, and mentally when our thoughts and feelings coincide with another's. If we are very lucky, we find both in the one relationship; but many never do.

I do not disparage the ego. We could not manage our earthly lives without it, and the ego has been used to achieve great things in the service of humankind. However, as depicted in the Buddhist ox-herding pictures from the Far East, the ego needs to be harnessed like the ox before the cart. When it is running out of control, especially when imagining itself to be under attack, the ego is highly dangerous. For instance, when the ego is attached to a piece of land, people are prepared to kill or die in the fight to own it. This happens when sovereignty is mistakenly being attributed to the material world, instead of understanding it to be a quality of the soul.

The Spiritual Self

According to the theoretical quantum physicist Amit Goswami, consciousness and matter arise simultaneously from what is called the 'collapse of the wave function'.[8] Out of a virtual wave of infinite *potentia*, a space-time domain is born (the physical universe) in which we find ourselves deposited, body and soul, on the little planet we call Earth. Yet we arrive recollecting hazily that we were *somewhere* before we took human form, as in these lines by William Wordsworth:[9]

> '...Not in entire forgetfulness,
> And not in utter nakedness,
> But trailing clouds of glory, do we come...'

Goswami's theory of monistic idealism describes the virtual wave function as containing all that ever was, is and shall be. However, since the virtual wave holds all *in potentia*, it does not contribute to the narrative of the mundane self. Instead, it feeds the immaterial soul, which retains the awareness of what it means to experience the absolute unity and perfection of the quantum realm.[10]

My intuition likewise told me that there was more to the universe than its constituent atoms, molecules, amino acids, carbon chains and so on. But what of the supreme presence that guides physical matter into its myriad forms and that manifests as consciousness? Eventually, I traded the 'bottom-up' perspective of psychoanalysis for the 'top-down vision' of a spiritual universe, a re-visioning that better answered the kind of questions I was asking.

In time, I came to appreciate that 'top-down' and 'bottom-up' are two sides of the same coin. Nevertheless, one side or other will usually appeal to a person more, for how we look at the world is highly subjective. 'We don't see things as they are; we see them as we are'.[11] This is perhaps just as well, since diversity is a great spur to discovery. Arguments are all very well, as long as they are not taken too seriously. I mean by this that if we identify with a thought, as the egoic mind likes to do, we may forget that we are not the thought but merely the one who dreamed it up, and then we may start proclaiming the thought

---

8. Goswami (1993).
9. *Ode: Intimations of Immortality from Recollections of Early Childhood*, stanza 5. See Wordsworth (2012).
10. In *Timaeus of Locri*, Plato prefigures the transpersonal significance of quantum mechanics when he writes: 'God [is] a circle whose centre is everywhere and circumference nowhere'.
11. A neat aphorism variously attributed to the Babylonian Talmud, G.T.W. Patrick, Henry Tomlinson, Anaïs Nin and Steven Covey!

to be 'the truth'.¹² The history of humanity is littered with the wreckage left by such proclamations.

Earlier, when paraphrasing William Blake, I remarked that the baby appears to see not *with* but *through* the eye. The soul is very much present but since the egoic self has not yet formed, there can be little exchange between them. Later in life, there is the prospect of a dialogue in which the soul can share its wisdom and compassion with the storm-tossed ego, now bereft of its complacency. Past life therapy, like other soul-centred approaches, can help to bring this about.

A Crisis of Modernity

The parlous state of the world today is the outcome of the unbridled action of the ego. Humanity suffers the consequences of the ego's territorial mentality, now being remorselessly acted out on the world stage. Will *Homo sapiens* ever be able to make the shift from separatism, arising from the ego's need to take, to unity based on the desire of the soul to give?¹³

My focus in this paper is on the soul perspective, and in particular how 'past lives' can help us to fulfil our human potential. To quote Marcel Proust, 'The only true voyage [...] would be not to visit strange lands but to possess other eyes'.¹⁴

Although the mundane self sees only the one journey from birth to death, the soul perspective that attracts me is seeing this life as a scene from a never-ending play, in which playwright, director, protagonist and audience are all projections of the one and same.¹⁵ The purpose of the drama, with its gamut of experiences and emotions of every kind, is to challenge us to become the best that we can be.

During childhood we are guided and restrained by our parents or else we should turn into little monsters. Parental influence contributes to the formation of the superego,¹⁶ held by Freud to be necessary for civilisation. The emerging ego has a hard time trying to find a

---

12. We go looking for, and generally find, the evidence that will affirm our worldview. Since nothing can be proven *not* to exist, the argument between material realism and metaphysics is likely to continue indefinitely.
13. See *Varieties of Love and the Near-Life Experience*, in Powell (2017).
14. Proust (2006: 657).
15. A metaphor that struck me as apt when I was training in psychodrama. See also *The Whole Patient*, this volume.
16. Freud's structural model of the psyche. For a concise summary, see Rycroft (1968: 160).

balance between the prohibitions of the superego and the clamour of instinctual demands. Compromises must be found if we are to reach adulthood, hopefully with some accomplishments, doing something useful, having a capacity for loving relationships and with a social conscience.

Human civilisation is, however, still very young. It has been said that if the timeline of Earth were to be compared with the height of the Empire State Building and its 102 floors, the past 5000 years would be no thicker than the paper covering one ceiling of one floor! It is hardly surprising that we still have dictatorships vying with democracies and that the currency of social exchange is more often power than love.

Given that there must be far more advanced civilisations than ours seeded throughout the universe, the human race is like the new kid on the block. The sci-fi portrayal of hostile extra-terrestrials is surely a paranoid projection of human fear and aggression. Who knows how many emergent life forms like ours go on to self-destruct? Only species that progress from conflict to collaboration could survive long term and duly take their place amongst stellar civilisations. It would appear that *Homo sapiens* has a long way to go.

Since the Abrahamic faiths make earthly death a one-off, there is no inbuilt means of a person continuing with their self-improvement. Given how far most of us have yet spiritually to travel, we might feel somewhat daunted. On the other hand, the prospect of reincarnation affords unlimited opportunity for further learning. According to the law of karma (cause and effect), every thought, word and deed is perfectly weighed in the balance and the life that we each are leading in the world today reflects our progress, such as it is, to date, and sets the stage for our future.

The Direct Experience

There is one more piece of the cosmic puzzle that I want to mention and it concerns the nature of the 'direct experience', also known as an awakening or epiphany. People who have had a direct experience do not report meeting spirits, travelling in other worlds, visiting past lives or indeed going anywhere. Yet the experience is deep and indelible, for in that heightened state of awareness everything is 'known'. There are no questions to ask and there is no meaning to be unpacked. Neither can the experience be truly conveyed in words. Words imply separation of subject and object and this is why words fail, since in the direct experience, observer and observed are one. The ancient Taoist text, the *Tao Te Ching*, begins with the lines:

'The Tao that can be told is not the eternal Tao,
The name that can be named is not the eternal name'.[17]

In Advaita Vedanta, we find the Sanskrit *neti neti*, meaning 'not this, not that', while Buddhists use the term *anatta* (not-self). The apophatic Western religious tradition speaks of the *via negativa*. None of these terms pretends to convey the richness of the direct experience.

Similarly, I cannot adequately describe the direct experience that happened to me some years ago. By way of analogy, I can say it was something like entering the projection room of a cosmic cinema showing an infinite number of films. I had stepped out of my own movie and gone behind the scenes. Here, beyond time and space, was perfect harmony like soundless music, and perfect movement, although everything was still. All was replete in itself.

Later, I came across the phrase 'multiplicity of virtual realities', which resonated deeply with me. When we exit our own movie, whether temporarily as in the out-of-body or near-death experience, or when re-living 'past lives', or irrevocably when we undergo bodily death, other movies await in which we play our part according to the agenda of the soul. Yet behind the dramas being projected on to myriad cosmic screens lies the Godhead, the ineffable source of all that was, is and ever shall be.

What Survives?

Edward Fitzgerald, who translated the *Rubáiyát*, considered Omar Khayyám to be an unrepentant Epicurean, raising a glass to the ephemeral moment – a defiant gesture in the face of oblivion. Yet Omar Khayyám is also believed to have studied Sufism and many quatrains are suffused with hints of eternal renewal:

'I sometimes think that never blows so red
That Rose as where some buried Caesar bled;
That every Hyacinth the Garden wears
Dropt in its Lap from some once lovely head.'

Will my individual consciousness continue when this particular movie ends? My ego would like this very much and indeed perhaps it will

---
17. Feng & English (1973).

be so. Some would say that since the Creator goes to such trouble to embody the spiritual self, it makes sense that our personal quotient of consciousness should be further developed and refined rather than disappearing, like raindrops falling on water.

Buddhists, on the other hand, believe our destiny is to merge with the universe, with new life arising from psychophysical aggregates called *skandhas* (form, sensation, perception, volition and consciousness). The chief objection in Buddhism to the notion of a unique and enduring soul is that since the *skandhas* are constantly changing, the self cannot be unchanging. Furthermore, since *skandhas* are transient, the self cannot be eternal and since they are diverse, the self cannot be unitary. This leads to the Buddhist notion of no-self.

My preferred view of the soul is not that in any way it should be fixed, but rather that it continually evolves as we journey through a multiplicity of virtual realities. There is a paradox here but not, I think, one that deters. Within domains of space-time, the universe is free to evolve and yet beyond all time and space, there can be no form, no movement and therefore nothing to evolve!

When I was a schoolboy and learning about angular velocity, I happened to notice a piece of fluff on the edge of an old style gramophone record moving past my eye at speed. Positioning it halfway to the centre, I could see that it travelled more slowly. Closer still to the centre, it was barely moving. Then I grasped that in the very centre, there must be a 'turning point' that stays perfectly still. Years later, I came across these memorable lines by T.S. Eliot:[18]

> 'At the still point of the turning world. Neither flesh nor fleshless;
> Neither from nor towards; at the still point, there the dance is,
> But neither arrest nor movement. And do not call it fixity,
> Where past and future are gathered. Neither movement from nor towards,
> Neither ascent nor decline. Except for the point, the still point,
> There would be no dance, and there is only the dance.'

I like to think that the direct experience takes us to the still point at the very centre. As for all the rest, we know it as life, seemingly confined to our familiar space-time locale, although very likely one among countless other locales.

Generally, we experience such life *de novo* but when a past life memory arises, we can make use of it to see better where we have come from, where we may be heading and what we need to learn – not only through re-visiting the life but also when it is over, with the clarity and

---

18. Eliot (1999).

forbearance of the spiritual self. From that vantage point, we are better able to see what the life's purpose may have been, with understanding, compassion and forgiveness not always within reach of the mundane self.

Past Life Memory

What is really happening to us when we engage with a past life? Some will argue the case for cryptomnesia (buried or forgotten memories). Others, in support of reincarnation, will cite the extensive field research of Ian Stevenson.[19]

I cannot know for sure whether the past lives I have experienced are evocations of my unconscious, were real lives lived by the same self I take myself to be today, or whether sympathetic resonance drew me to a life once lived and which became 'mine', much as a visitor might enter a room for an hour or two and make themselves at home – in which case I could as well say that the past life 'lived me'. I do know, however, that the therapeutic effect is profound.

I am not going to go into the technique of past life therapy in this paper but for those interested in the 'how to', the Jungian analyst Roger Woolger has written a full and lively account, including many case studies.[20] Nevertheless, I earlier alluded to one golden rule. When working with a past life, especially when the ending has been traumatic, it is essential the therapist enables the client fully to complete the life by going through, and beyond, bodily death. If stopped short in the midst of painful death memories, the experience may leave a person further traumatised, whereas going through and beyond death brings release from the travails of bodily existence and the opportunity to find healing.

From the place of the afterlife (or *bardo*, as it is known in Tibetan Buddhism) the therapist actively works with the client to explore the meaning of that life and to complete any unfinished business that remains. As the ego yields to the wisdom of the soul, deep learning takes place. This way the body does not have to die before a person gets the lessons they need! Furthermore, within a short time, you are back in the world with your new insights on board and ready to put learning into practice.

This is best illustrated by letting past life narrative speak for itself. The three that follow are from among those that I experienced when training in past life regression.

---

19. Tucker (2005).
20. Woolger (1988).

An Embittered Death[21]

I find myself in Nantes, in France.[22] It is the 16th century and I am a miller, with a wife and two daughters. I am at home when the door suddenly bursts open and soldiers arrest me. I am perfunctorily tied up, thrown onto a cart and taken to the jail. There a military tribunal arraigns me. I am accused of supporting a civil insurrection by supplying grain to rebel forces. I am innocent and protest, but given no chance to defend myself. Instead, I am pronounced guilty of treason and thrown into a dungeon where I am chained to the stone floor. There I suffer unceasing privation – there is no one to speak with, disgusting food is passed wordlessly to me once a day and no one comes to see me. I lose track of time and I lose all hope. Years pass, and there is nothing but my suffering. I have been abandoned. Worst of all, my wife never once comes to see me.

In the therapy session, we move forward year by year until I come to the last hour of the last day of my life. I see that my leg is gangrenous where the chain has cut into the flesh. I begin to lose consciousness. Then suddenly I am looking down at my body and there is no more pain. I turn towards the light and leave. I find myself in a place outdoors, bathed in light that I have not seen in years. There is blessed freedom, yet I am aware that I still harbour a deep grievance.

Now the therapist asks me whom I might wish to meet. I immediately say, with great bitterness, 'Not my wife, for she deserted me'. The therapist suggests it could be important to tell her how I feel and grudgingly I consent. I wait a short while (time in the *bardo* is fluid) and then she too crosses over. She catches sight of me and runs towards me with joy. I feel deep anger towards her and prepare to push her away. 'It's you', she cries. 'I came to the prison every day to see you, for all those years, and they never let me in!' My eyes fill with tears and I am flooded with remorse. I am deeply ashamed of my lack of trust and I beg for her forgiveness. She embraces me and we are together again. We wait there in each other's arms until our two children come across at the conclusion of their lives, and so are united in love once more as family.

This session vividly brought home to me the importance of maintaining faith in the goodness of love. Without it, I should be ensnared in endless suffering, for a broken heart is worse than a physical affliction. It also shows that when we cross over into the *bardo*, we carry with us the powerful imprint of the last emotion before death. If reconciliation

---

21. The past lives 'An Embittered Death' and 'When All Seems Lost' are also described in *Death and Soul Consciousness*, in Powell (2017).
22. Curiosity prompted me to look up the French wars of religion between the Catholics and the Protestant Huguenots. A truce, the Edict of Nantes, was finally declared by Henry IV in 1598.

and forgiveness are not sought and found, the negative imprint carries over into the next life. There it will need facing again, for the wound remains open until healing can take place.

A Life Abandoned

I am living as a wealthy squire in 17th-century England. I have a beautiful country house, a lovely wife, Elizabeth, and a son and daughter. Then, while the children are still young, my beloved wife catches a chill and dies of a fever. I am distraught. I withdraw from the world, become distant from my children and pace around my house and gardens like a ghost. I cannot forgive God for taking my wife from me and I lose my faith. I never recover from this melancholy and the years pass silently and monotonously. When I finally become ill, I have no desire to recover. Instead, I welcome death, which comes to me one day while I am staring at sunlight streaming through the stained glass window in my chamber.

The first person to meet me on the other side is my wife Elizabeth, looking in the bloom of youth. I can hardly believe my eyes. There is great joy in our meeting! Then, with awful clarity, I see that in my anger and despair I threw away the precious gift of my life. All I had needed to do was be patient and wait for us to be re-united. I had been given our children to love and cherish, and I could have treasured the memory of my wife through my love for them. Instead, I had been victim to my grief and it had eventually poisoned me.

The common strand between these two examples of past lives is that of enforced separation and loss. It is inevitable that life brings suffering. What is crucial is how we meet it and ensure that it does not destroy our humanity. I was being shown never to turn my back on life and love.[23]

When All Seems Lost

I am a young man, the son of a cobbler, living in a village on the coast in southwest England in the 18th century. Engaged to be married, I am well liked and in the best of health. Yet it is not enough for me that I have loving parents, a sweetheart and an honest job working with my

---

23. Viktor Frankl, who survived four Nazi death camps between 1942 and 1945, writes of the realisation that came to him in the midst of his suffering as he recalled his wife's image. 'Then I grasped the meaning of the greatest secret that human poetry and human thought and belief have to impart: The salvation of man is through love and in love'. Frankl (1946: 37).

father. Like many of the young men around, I am lining my pockets with sovereigns by joining a local group of smugglers bringing in French brandy from across the Channel.

Then, one evening, disaster strikes. The boat is due to land with its cargo and I have been put ashore in an adjacent cove to go up the cliff path and rendezvous with the lookout. As I reach the cliff top, I hear musket fire from the cove below. The militia have been lying in wait and are slaughtering the crew. I flee, and within a few hours have travelled farther afield than ever before in my whole life. I am safe for the moment, but what should I do now? I dare not go back home, I know no one and I have no money.

Either I will starve or I must steal, and so begins my life as a thief. In time, I graduate to living the squalid life of a highwayman holding up stagecoaches. I am caught in a downward spiral and I know that at some time, I will probably end up a murderer as well as a thief.

One day, when stopping a stagecoach, I find myself staring at a half-dozen muskets all trained on me. The militia, hiding within, have found their man. I am bound and taken to the nearest town. In the morning, a judge finds me guilty to be hanged. A noose is put round my neck as I stand on a cart, which is driven away. I hang there until I die.

I move away from my body but find I can't leave the gibbet from which my lifeless body still hangs. People come to stare, crows peck out my eyes and my body begins to rot. Then some soldiers cut my body down and throw it into a pit of lime. I still cannot leave that place. My desolation is profound. I feel deep shame for having wasted my whole life for a few sovereigns. My parents had been proud of me. I had let them down, myself too, and all those dear to me.

My therapist now asks me to see if there might be someone to come to my aid and accompany me from there towards the light. I wait for what seems a long time but no one comes. Eventually the therapist reminds me that I could always pray for help. I hardly dare do so, for I cannot imagine I deserve forgiveness. Finally I call out, 'God, please help me'. Immediately, a light appears to which I am powerfully drawn and I soar away from that dreadful place.

This past life taught me an important lesson: it really is possible to make such a mess of earthly life that a person must thereafter live out the consequence of their folly. Yet it also brought home to me that it is never too late to ask for help – without having to die first!

In Conclusion

Jacob Moreno, the founder of psychodrama, once said that psychodrama is a place where you can learn from your mistakes without being punished. I would add that past life therapy is a place where you can re-visit your worst ordeals, witness the consequences and, most importantly, find the healing for which the soul yearns. Then you walk right back into your life to see if you can put to good use what you have learned.

This world is a melting pot of the good, the bad and the indifferent, which makes it a great place either for self improvement or self-destruction. Presumably this is why we come here, to make of it Hell or Heaven according to our will. Thus far, it seems that the human race has not yet sufficiently evolved to be moved collectively by the love, wisdom and guidance of the soul. As a species, we behave as recklessly as putting a child behind the wheel of a car and saying, 'Go, drive!' There have been some fearful smashes in human history with doubtless more to come.

Nevertheless, from the soul perspective the only fatality is that of the physical body. This comment does not make light of abuse, torture or the many sufferings that afflict humankind, but is to remind us that from the vantage point of the journey of the soul, every incarnation brings the opportunity to grow in wisdom, understanding and compassion. Like children, we need loving guidance and we have had some great souls here on Earth as our exemplars. Yet we cannot run before we walk, and those great souls will have endured their struggles too.

Why bother with past lives at all? Why not leave it to the greater scheme of things to sort this out without pitching in with our good intentions? This is largely what happens in any case. Yet it seems to me that if we chance upon a past life, the important thing is to use it to learn and grow.

Aside from occasional déjà vu, we generally meet life as though experiencing it for the very first time. This ensures we take it seriously – as the maxim goes, life is not a rehearsal! Yet if we glimpse, whether by chance or design, other times and other places where we have travelled before, it serves to remind us that we are spiritual beings on a human path, with the opportunity to transcend the confines of the ego, overcome the captivity of the past and open the way to a new future.

Nearly one millennium ago, Omar Khayyám penned this poetic yet resigned quatrain:

> 'For in and out, above, about, below,
> 'Tis nothing but a Magic Shadow-show
> Play'd in a Box whose candle is the Sun
> Round which we Phantom Figures come and go.'

I have no hesitation in bequeathing 'nothing but' to Richard Dawkins[24] and his popular brand of material realism. The exploration of soul consciousness shows us that this magic shadow-show is of our own making. What may appear to be a circular motion is nothing less than a spiral that takes us beyond our wildest dreams.

References

Baron-Cohen, S., Tager-Flusberg, H. & Cohen, D. (1999) *Understanding Other Minds: Perspectives from Autism and Cognitive Neuroscience.* Oxford University Press.
Blake, W. (1917) The Everlasting Gospel. In *The Oxford Book of English Mystical Verse* (eds D. Nicholson & A. Lee). Clarendon Press.
Dawkins, R. (1976) *The Selfish Gene.* Oxford University Press.
Eliot, T.S. (1999) Burnt Norton. In *Four Quartets.* Faber & Faber.
Feng, G.F. & English, J. (trans.) (1973) *Lao Tsu: Tao Te Ching* (section 1). Wildwood House.
Fitzgerald, E. (1989) *The Rubáiyát of Omar Khayyám.* Collins.
Frankl, V. (1946) *Man's Search for Meaning.* Reprinted [2000]. Beacon Press.
Goswami, A. (1993) *The Self-Aware Universe: How Consciousness Creates the Material World.* Tarcher/Putnam.
Powell, A. (2017) *The Ways of the Soul: A Psychiatrist Reflects. Essays on Life, Death and Beyond.* Muswell Hill Press.
Proust, M. (2006) *Remembrance of Things Past,* vol. 2 (transl. C.K. Scott Moncrieff & S. Hudson). Wordsworth Edition.
Rycroft, C. (1968) *A Critical Dictionary of Psychoanalysis.* Penguin.
Tucker, J. (2005) *Life before Life: A Scientific Investigation of Children's Memories of Previous Lives.* St. Martin's Press.
Woolger, R. (1988) *Other Lives, Other Selves: A Jungian Psychotherapist Discovers Past Lives.* Bantam Books.
Wordsworth, W. (2012) *Lyrical Ballads by William Wordsworth.* Forgotten Books.

---

24. Prolific author, professed atheist and formerly University of Oxford's Professor for Public Understanding of Science, Dawkins first came to prominence with his 1976 book *The Selfish Gene.* Dawkins contends that religious faith is a delusion.

6

Soul-Centred Psychotherapy

The term soul-centred psychotherapy encompasses a range of psycho-spiritual approaches, all of which place the emphasis on that repository of wisdom and love found in every human being – the soul. Before giving examples of my own practice of soul-centred therapy, I would like to set out my understanding of 'spirituality', 'soul' and 'spirit', words that are all profoundly expressive of the inner life.

I have described spirituality as the experience of deeply felt meaning and purpose in life and a sense of wholeness and belonging that brings harmony and peace. For some, this finds fulfilment in loving human relationships, while for others it must admit the relationship with God as the ultimate source of love. As a transpersonal quest, spirituality entails searching for answers about the infinite that lies beyond earthly life, and can be particularly important at times of illness, loss, bereavement and death.[1]

The spiritual longing for wholeness permeates body, soul and spirit. With the body, we celebrate the gift of life in eating, drinking, making love and bearing children – a primeval spiritual impulse that seeks to merge two into one. When we are attuned to soul, we see that we are mirrored in each other and that all humanity is one family. When we align ourselves with spirit, we move beyond personal identity, opening ourselves to the transcendent in humility and awe.

By the word 'spirit' I refer to the limitless and unbounded consciousness that energises *all that is*, both latent and manifest. I use the word 'soul' to describe the manifestation of spirit through form. In this sense, at the level of a vibration of atoms, a pebble on the beach can be said to have a soul. In the plant kingdom, soul takes the form of a collective

Paper prepared for the annual conference of the Transpersonal Section of the British Psychological Society, Scarborough, September 2009.

---

1. As also given in *Spirituality and Psychiatry – Crossing the Divide*, this volume.

sentient field. In the animal kingdom, soul acquires awareness (dogs and cats possess 'awareness' much as we do). Soul in the human species has advanced to the stage of self-awareness – a privilege that opens the door to heaven or hell on Earth, depending on our intentions.

Self-awareness bestows on us our unique individuality. Whether individuality, once acquired, is preserved for eternity, or whether our ultimate destination is to merge with the energy of all that is, none of us can know for sure. However, given that our universe exists among myriad domains of space-time, it seems very likely to me that we move from one such domain to another at points of transition: altered states of consciousness such as out-of-body and near-death experiences, meditation, dreaming and, most of all, what we know as death.

Because our sense perception attunes us to physical reality, we forget that everything is one sea of energy, mysteriously coalescing into form and then dissolving back into formlessness, and that the physical body is but a temporary condensation of molecules. In contrast, the soul, having no mass, is untouched by entropy and the laws of physics. Experiencing this life as precious but ephemeral, the soul views the death of the body with equanimity.

The ego, on the other hand, arises from the need to grow and survive as an individual life form in the physical world. Consequently, the ego fears death, indeed tries to deny it, since it dreads the prospect of obliteration. Yet the ego is necessary, especially for the first half of life, when we desire to make our mark on the world – an impression the ego likes to think is going to last. The soul, however, calmly watching as the seasons of life flow by, is on hand to offer help, especially in the later years, when we are obliged to harvest what earlier we sowed.

Soul and ego must live together; without the ego there would be no journey for the soul to take, and without the soul, the human species would be destined to remain forever the most destructive species on Earth.[2] Keeping the bigger picture in view enables me to remain hopeful. We are being schooled, for our improvement, in the law of cause and effect (known in the East as karma), which teaches – some say over many lifetimes – that we are accountable for our every thought, word and deed. The human race is still a very juvenile species and we have not yet learned how to stop acting on the impulses of the ego and heed the soul. Nevertheless, if *Homo sapiens* survives long enough to live up to its name, a brighter future awaits.

As a psychiatrist, I came to soul-centred therapy via a roundabout route that included psychoanalysis, group analysis, psychodrama and

---

2. It has been estimated that warfare in the 20th century resulted in more than 130 million military and civilian deaths. See Leitenberg (2006).

the work of Carl Jung, and later I went on to study healing and other transpersonal therapies. My aim here is to illustrate some of the many ways in which it is possible to enlist the help of the soul in clinical practice. I shall group the illustrations according to the approach taken, starting with three examples of 'engaging' the soul.[3]

Searching for the Soul

Christine was chronically depressed. Throughout childhood, she never felt valued. Academic success had temporarily bolstered her self-esteem, but later, when a personal relationship failed, this fell apart. Her emotions froze over and she became profoundly withdrawn.

> Christine had described her depression as a black cave. I invited her to close her eyes, 'go inside' and report with what she could find. After some minutes, she found a pair of steel handcuffs, then a rope and an iron chain. I pressed her to go on looking. After what seemed an eternity, her expression changed to one of concern and I asked her what she had found. It was a little puppy in a dark corner. I suggested she pick it up and hold it to her. With her eyes still closed, she cradled the puppy. What could she feel? She replied that she could feel the puppy's love for her. I urged her to let her own love flow to this puppy and she began to cry. I encouraged her to find an image for her emotion and she chose a golden heart.

The process can be understood psychologically as the puppy symbolising the child Christine. She rediscovers and nurtures this child-self with which she had lost touch, and in doing so discovers that she still has the capacity for love. On the transpersonal level, Christine is reclaiming her soul that had been lost to view in the darkness of her childhood.

Treasuring the Soul

Carol's history had been one of terrible abuse and for years, she had taken refuge in alcohol. During the first interview, I encouraged her to look inside herself and tell me what she found there.

> What Carol saw was 'her heart beating so hard it could burst'. When I asked her what she wanted to do with it, she said she would put it to rest

---

3. The case studies included here were recorded prior to the Data Protection Act 1998. Some are also cited in *The Ways of the Soul*, Powell (2017).

in a silk-lined coffin, adding, 'Only death will bring it peace'. But then, after a moment, the heart transformed into a little whirligig of energy. It would not be trapped but flew about the room, so she released it and watched it fly away.

On this occasion, Carol was not ready or able to take up the offer of therapy, which would also have meant giving up alcohol. However, four years later she came to see me again, having faced up to her drinking in the meantime.

This time, when Carol closed her eyes and went within, she found a treasure chest. I asked if she might pick up the treasure chest and she put it under her arm. Passing through an archway, she found herself in a sandy desert, by a pool of water and some trees. She sat by the water, resting peacefully, and said with a sigh, 'This is for me!' (All her life she has rushed around trying to please others.) Did she want to drink? She drank deeply of the cool fresh water. Now where did she need to go? She immediately found herself back home, still holding the treasure chest, studded with jewels and very beautiful. She placed it on the floor in the middle of the room.

The first time Carol came, she could not engage creatively with her soul. Peace only equated with death. Yet images of the soul are incapable of death – hence the whirligig. On the second occasion, Carol showed that she was ready for therapy, which was subsequently offered.

Soul to Soul

Rosemary came to see me several years after her teenage daughter Tessa had attempted suicide, which had left the girl with severe brain damage. Rosemary felt deeply responsible and the torment of her grief was immense. She could barely bring herself to visit her once-lovely daughter, who now lay immobile with severe contractures. In a session that followed a rare visit to the nursing home, she raged, 'I cannot bear seeing what she has turned into'.

> I had been struck by a comment of Rosemary's, that she dreaded going to see Tessa because as she approached the room and even before opening the door, Tessa, who normally lay silent and motionless, would start to make loud moaning noises. Did Tessa somehow sense that this was her mother visiting?
>
> It seemed to me that for healing to take place, it was important that Rosemary found a way to face her daughter. I suggested that when entering the room, Rosemary fixed her gaze only on Tessa's eyes, making sure not to look at her body while she drew near. We took time to rehearse

this in the session. When Rosemary next visited, she went right up to Tessa, making sure to look only in her eyes. Tessa then stopped moaning and began to fixate on her mother's eyes. Rosemary found herself cradling her daughter and telling her that she loved her and would be coming again. One year later, Tessa was able to communicate a little with the help of a clock alphabet. She was now trying to crawl and surgery was being considered for treatment of her contractures.

This example bears out the proverb, found the world over, that 'the eye is the mirror of the soul'.

Soul Retrieval

Soul retrieval is a feature of shamanic healing in which a soul that has fallen under a malign influence needs freeing and returning to its rightful place. In the following example, this approach is used to help a person find release from the terrors of her childhood.

> Sally, in her mid-fifties, was suffering from treatment-resistant depression. Her problems had begun in early childhood, which had been blighted with insecurity. When she was seven, she fell into the hands of a fundamentalist schoolteacher, Miss Edwards, who terrified the child with threats of hell and damnation. Sally had recurring visions of flames licking around her bed and the red face of the devil would appear at night and in her dreams. In adulthood, Sally seemed to overcome her fears, but following major surgery, which left her body scarred, she once again succumbed to these visions, living from day to day in a state of sheer panic.
>
> First, I encouraged Sally to visualise her soul. She located it inside her chest but as a feeble thing, not much more than a glimmer of light. I asked her to look carefully to see if there were any strands or cords running out from it into the darkness. She found such a cord, so I urged her to follow it and see where it led. After a moment she looked up and said she could see Miss Edwards, looking very old but as fierce as ever, holding the end of the cord tightly in her hand.
>
> I then had a frank discussion with Miss Edwards, speaking with her through the agency of Sally. Miss Edwards insisted that what she did was right, the child had to be controlled and if she instilled fear in her, it was for her own good. I pointed out that instead of helping it had only led to a lifetime of misery and torment. Is this what Miss Edwards as a Christian really intended? She faltered and I pressed home my advantage. She herself would now be nearing the end of her life and soon facing her Maker. How will she be judged? Then Miss Edwards became fearful. She hadn't intended harm and she hoped God would have pity on her. I put it to her that she could start making amends right now by letting go of Sally's soul and giving it back to her. Miss Edwards

agreed and let go of the cord. I asked Sally to draw it back into herself, after which we spent some time on healing.

Following the session, Sally reported that the red devil had lost his power over her. The next step would be to help Sally find compassion for that child who had lived with so much fear.

In psychodynamic therapy, terms such as projection and introjection are employed metaphorically. In contrast, the shamanic tradition treats projection and introjection as palpable, energetic realities. The argument about what really is going on will doubtless continue, but what matters much more to the patient is finding relief from suffering.

The next three accounts show the power of the transpersonal realm in enabling relief from bereavement that cannot be found in ordinary waking life.

Reunion of Souls

Joan came to see me about a year after the death of her husband Ted, whom she had nursed through a long and debilitating illness. They had been together 40 years and her loss left her grief-stricken. She continually felt Ted's presence around the house, yet the awareness brought only pain.

> I asked Joan if she thought there could be an afterlife. Yes, she thought there might be, but how could that help her now? I then put it to Joan that we could try to make contact with Ted in a way that may help bring her peace of mind.
>
> At my suggestion, she shut her eyes, relaxed, and was encouraged to see if she could 'find' Ted wherever he might be. After a couple of minutes, a faint smile played on her lips. I asked Joan what she saw. She replied that she could see Ted in his cricket whites, playing cricket and looking very fit and happy. I remarked that he seemed to be enjoying a game of heavenly cricket! Joan's smile widened and she added that cricket had been Ted's great passion. Then a look of deep sadness passed across her face. I asked whether she would like to speak with Ted. She nodded, so I suggested she walk up to him and see what might happen. After a moment, Joan said that she was now next to Ted and that he had put his arm around her. What was he saying? He was saying 'Don't worry; everything is going to be all right.' I asked Joan to look around her. Was anyone else present? Then she saw her deceased sister and parents there, smiling and waving to her.

Being able to see death not as an ending but as a transition helped Joan to resume life with hope and expectation.

A Soul that was Never Born

Grace came with a depression that could be traced back to her earlier decision to have an abortion. She had been a young, single woman who found herself pregnant after a brief relationship. She felt sure at the time that it would be in everyone's best interests to end the pregnancy, so she sought medical advice and a planned termination was performed. Her physical recovery was uneventful, life moved on and after some time she entered a new relationship that led to marriage. The couple tried for a child, but Grace did not fall pregnant. She became depressed, finding herself thinking back to the earlier termination of pregnancy, which she had always kept secret. She began to feel that her failure to conceive now was a punishment for 'getting rid' of her baby.

> In the session, as we explored her feelings about the termination, Grace began to cry. I asked her if she had ever wanted to talk with her unborn baby and she nodded. I said that we might do that now if she wished. Again, she nodded, so I handed her a pillow, asked her to cradle it in her arms, close her eyes and picture the baby she was holding. She began sobbing. 'What do you need to say to your baby?' I urged. Grace burst out, 'What have I done? I'm so sorry for what I did to you'. I said to Grace, 'Now let your baby speak through you', and I asked the baby, 'What did Grace do to you?' The words that came back were shocking. The baby answered, 'It was terrible. I was just lying there and then something came in and I was torn to pieces'.[4]
>
> Grace was racked with remorse. 'What else do you want Grace to know?' I asked the baby. 'Please stop crying', said the baby through her. 'It was all over very quickly, and I'm fine now'. I then said to the baby, 'Do you know that Grace cannot forgive herself for what she did?' The baby answered her, 'You did the best you could at the time. And it was very nice being in you, even though I never got born. Don't blame yourself. I'm fine now, it's true'. I asked Grace if she wanted to say anything more to the baby. She cried 'I'm so sorry, and I miss you and I think about you so much'. The baby answered her, 'It's only for now – we'll see each other again soon'. I asked Grace to take some time in silence to be with her baby. As she sat rocking and holding the pillow, she gradually quietened. Then I asked her and the baby to say goodbye to each other for the present. Before she left, Grace decided to tell her husband what had happened. I do not know if she subsequently became pregnant but I hope her chances will have improved.

---

4. In a termination of pregnancy, the foetus, as doctors call it, is sucked out with a vacuum tube. It is not widely known that in the course of doing so, the foetus is dismembered.

Souls may be together for only a short time, as with children who die young or who never reach their day of birth. Yet every meeting of souls is deeply meaningful and deserves to be honoured and, on occasions, mourned with love.

A Soul Dream

My patient, John, had been born into circumstances of great deprivation. Fortunately, he was saved from a life in social care by being taken in, aged four, by a neighbour, Bob, who from that time on was father in all but name.

The boy grew into a man and made good. He married, had a family and moved away. Yet he often went back to see Bob, now ageing and alone but fiercely independent. Then the time came when Bob grew so frail that his neighbours had to come in and start washing and caring for him. Bob couldn't bear it. One day he got himself upstairs to the spare bedroom, lay down with his cap on his head as always, swallowed a lot of tablets and died.

My patient was devastated at the news. He kept dreaming Bob was still alive only to wake up and find him gone. He fell into a severe depression.

> John then told me that just before attending this consultation, something had happened which had 'knocked him for six'. He had dreamed again of Bob but this was different. In the dream, he 'knew' for the first time that Bob was dead. Yet there was Bob, sitting across from him, large as life, cap on head, just the way he always sat. My patient asked him outright, 'Bob, are you dead?' Bob answered him as direct as ever, 'Yes!' His next question to Bob was, 'Is there life after death?' Another emphatic 'Yes', came right back. Then he challenged Bob head on. 'Prove it to me!' Bob pulled out a book that looked like a Bible with detailed drawings in it and, sure enough, the proof was all there.
>
> Then John awoke. All day he could intensely feel Bob's presence. He found his emotions welling up and although it was very painful, he could say to me in that first meeting 'I know I'm getting better'.

The Soul Remembers

Sometimes entering the transpersonal realm will take a person from one life to another, as in the next two examples of 'past life' memories.[5]

---

5. See also *Past Life Memory – A Key to Understanding the Self?*, this volume.

Peter, aged twenty-seven, came to see me with a water phobia. Having been a good swimmer and with no evident neurotic traits, he was travelling on a small ferry when he suffered a severe panic attack. He had been looking over the side of the boat at the time when the thought came to him that if he were to fall overboard, he would be swept away and drowned. Worst of all, no one would ever know what had happened to him.

Going into Peter's personal history revealed no obvious cause for this acute episode. I asked him to close his eyes and re-live the scene, this time imagining falling into the water. Peter's body immediately began jerking and thrashing about. I asked him, 'What's happening?' Peter cried out, 'I can't get free. I'm drowning'. I then instructed him to go back in time to just before the moment of drowning. Suddenly he cried out, 'We've been rammed and water's coming in the boat'. 'Why can't you get free?' 'I'm chained to the boat!'

I took Peter forward in time to the moment of drowning. His struggling movements became weaker and he went limp. What was happening now? 'I'm leaving my body, I'm rising up through the water and I'm going higher, up into the sky.' 'What can you see?' 'There's a bright light, I want to go there.' I said, 'Before you leave, look back on this life you just lived and tell me about yourself and how old you are'. 'I'm 27' he said, and told the story of a young man fighting in the Greco-Persian wars, who had spent the last two years of his life as a slave oarsman on a Greek trireme. During a naval battle with the Persians, the ship had gone down with all on board. The young man's wife and children 'would never know what had happened to him'.

By way of intense emotional arousal – what is called an 'affect bridge' – Peter had slipped into a 'past life'. The process can be understood on different levels, from the psychological to the transpersonal. What is not in question is that such soul dramas can have an immediate and lasting therapeutic effect.

Healing for Two Souls

Alice was a 43-year-old woman who came with a 10-year history of sarcoidosis, an autoimmune disease that was causing her to go blind. She was increasingly reliant on her husband, John, to care for her. Theirs was a loving marriage and she said of him with a smile, 'He was a good catch!' Alice's loss of sight was challenging her to try to make sense of her misfortune. Recently she had heard about past life regression and wanted to see if it could provide any clue.

> The sarcoidosis had begun with blinding headaches. In the session, we went back to that time when she lay exhausted and crying, holding her head in her hands in a darkened room.

I asked Alice to find words for the terrible pain in her head. If her headache could speak, what would it say? She cried out, 'Let me alone. Let me be free.' I suggested she give in to the longing and see where it took her. Her face relaxed and she lay with her eyes closed and a smile on her lips. At once, she found herself lazing in the warm, calm water of a tropical ocean. I asked her to look around. She could see the sandy shore some way off and beyond that, dense vegetation covering the lower slopes of distant mountains. Next, I asked her to look down at her body. She said with astonishment, 'I'm… like a fish.' Then she exclaimed, 'No, not a fish, I'm a dolphin!' Her expression was one of intense pleasure. I asked if there were any other dolphins nearby. It transpired that this young dolphin had disobeyed her parents and had swum off on her own.

I then asked her to go forward in time to the next important thing that happened. She found herself lying on the sand, unable to move (Alice's body started making ineffectual jerking movements on the couch). I asked her to check her body, and she became aware of a large hole in her side. Now tears began to trickle down her cheeks. There was no pain but her strength was ebbing. She looked up and could see the prow of a boat a few feet away. Standing on it and staring down at her was a fisherman with painted face and body, holding a spear in his hand. Then the boat slid away. As darkness fell, she grew calm. Suddenly she found herself rising up into the sky and looking down, without emotion or regret, at the lifeless body of the dolphin on the beach.

Did this soul need to face the fisherman who had killed her with his spear? At first, she was reluctant, saying 'It wasn't his fault. He never killed another dolphin'. Then she agreed that it could be important. So, she 'waited' there for a while until his turn came to die and he crossed over. Now she could see the fisherman coming closer. Involuntarily, she found herself going forward and embracing him. I asked her if she recognised him. 'Of course, it's my husband John', Alice said, beginning to laugh and cry at the same time. 'He caught me and this time I've caught him. We are together and he is here to take care of me!'

As in the previous example, going through and beyond death is important, for otherwise, far from being therapeutic, the session could intensify the fear of dying. Frequently, in past life therapy there is unfinished business to attend to after leaving the body and before the soul leaves to go to the light. The insights gained give both solace and a deeper understanding of the current life situation.

Release for an Earthbound Spirit

Sometimes, as the next two case studies illustrate, the past impacts on the present not from a 'past life' but because the spirit of a deceased person has remained effectively stuck and unable to move on. In such cases, the therapist is working to free both their patient and the earth-bound spirit.

> Pat came for help having suffered from depression for many years. Since childhood, she longed for approval but felt she could never please. Her mother would mock and belittle her and Pat was often full of anger that she never dared express.
>
> When her mother died, Pat heaved a sigh of relief thinking she could now get on with her own life. But she found she could not, for her mother's presence was all around and she still seemed to hear her scorning her. Feeling possessed by her mother, as she herself put it, Pat had become suicidal.
>
> I said to Pat that suicide would resolve nothing and that we needed to find a way to help the two of them separate. I invited her to confront her mother in death as she had not been able to in life, with Pat using an empty chair to visualise her mother face-to-face. For the first time she was able to deliver a few home truths and told her mother it was time she got off her back.
>
> I now asked Pat to sit in the empty chair and reverse roles with mother. Mum came straight back, saying she had no intention of stopping! She enjoyed hanging around Pat and in any case, she had nowhere else to go.
>
> I asked Mum, through Pat, about her life that had just ended and I learned that her own mother had rejected her from an early age. She resolved to escape from home and took the first man she could to help her get away. However, finding herself pregnant when she was 17 ended her hopes of a career and tied her to a man she did not love. Her daughter Pat became the life-long target of her resentment.
>
> I explained to the mother how 'moving on' would help her find freedom and happiness and to look around for someone she knew, who had already crossed over, to accompany her along the way. To begin with nobody appeared, so I urged her to look for just one person in her whole life that had shown her kindness. After a long pause, she remembered a Mrs Cox, a nurse who had stayed with the mother's family for a time, and who made a real fuss over her when she had been a little girl. As Pat's mother recalled Mrs Cox, her face softened and I asked her to try to find her. Then she smiled and said she could now see her, looking just the way she did all those years ago. I asked her to take Mrs Cox's hand and walk towards the light. There was no further protest and she left with her friend. When this was over, Pat looked emotionally drained but at peace. She went back to her own chair and said, 'It feels that she has really gone, for the first time'.

The psychodramatic encounter helped Pat to ventilate her feelings more powerfully than by telling me *about* mother. In mother's place, Pat could experience first-hand the unhappiness that underlay her mother's bitterness. With greater understanding Pat no longer felt in thrall to her mother, and in participating in her mother's spirit release she was put in touch with her own compassion, important for her own healing.

Suicide and Spirit Attachment

Jan came to see me complaining of feeling depressed and *'not herself'*. Taking an antidepressant had helped but she was still not herself. I was struck by her use of the phrase.

Going into Jan's background, I learned that shortly before her symptoms started, a close friend had taken her life in Jan's home, having been staying there while my patient was away on holiday.

> Remembering how she had twice said she was 'not herself', I asked Jan if she had the feeling of 'someone else' when she came back home. She replied that she hadn't wanted to say in case I thought she was mad, but every time she went into the house, she had the physical sensation of her friend being right there in the room with her.
>
> Taking this at face value, I asked Jan if she would like me to invite the spirit of her deceased friend to the consultation to see if we could find out more about what was going on. Jan was willing, so I asked her to close her eyes, tune in to her friend and try letting her friend speak through her.
>
> Her friend 'came through' and went on to express deep regret at having taken her life. Suicide had solved nothing. She remained unhappy, lonely, and seeking comfort. I explained that staying on was having a bad effect on my patient, and was not helping herself either. She apologised. 'If only I had known', she said, 'what I know now. I was facing the biggest challenge of my life and I went and messed it up. I feel even worse than I did before'. I said I was sure other opportunities would be given her. She was very relieved to hear this and we talked more about her hopes for another chance at life. When she agreed that she was ready to move on, I asked her to look for 'the light'. She exclaimed, 'Yes, I can see it!', and left at once. Immediately, Jan felt the burden of oppression lift from her and it did not return.

Given that many faith traditions view suicide as a sin with dire consequences, this account holds two important messages. Firstly, no judgement is passed, except that of self-recrimination. Secondly, there is always the opportunity to learn from experience – and to do better next time.

'Demons', too, have Souls

In the Christian tradition, the ministry of deliverance is asked to take on cases of spirit possession. Similarly in Islam, interference by *jinn* may be dealt with by an imam. From time to time, spirit release therapists also find themselves treating cases of what appears to be demonic possession.[6]

> Janet, in her mid-twenties, had been depressed for many years. Her problems went back to an abusive relationship in her teens. Soon after, she developed chronic pelvic pain, for which she was now being told a hysterectomy might be needed.
>
> I asked Janet to go within, to 'scan' her body and tell me what she saw there. Right away, she described 'a nasty dark red thing' attached to her womb. I invited it to speak and it explained, through Janet, that it had been there since Janet was seventeen. It was belligerent and boastful, saying it had made her ill and wasn't finished yet – it was going to give her cancer. When she heard this, Janet exclaimed out loud, 'It's a demon!'
>
> She was anxious to free herself from this thing, so I suggested she visualise angels enclosing the 'demon' in a bubble of light. At once it cried out in fear, 'Stop, I'm going to burn!' I pointed out that it was already trapped by the light, so it had better take refuge in the darkness within itself. I urged it to go deeper and deeper, and after a while, it said with astonishment that it could see a light. The next moment it cried out in wonder, saying 'This feels so good, I feel so warm and nice!' Then it went on to say with great remorse, 'What have I done? I have caused such pain and misery!' I said that only by going into the light would it find forgiveness and the opportunity for redemption. It couldn't wait to leave!

This transformation of 'negative' energy is an important part of spirit release therapy. We can see the 'demon' as being just that, an attached entity, or we could regard it as a split-off aspect of the unconscious psyche. From the clinical standpoint, the important thing is to decide when to work for integration and when to go for removal. In this case, the energetic complex was treated as a spirit attachment and released into the light. However, further therapy would help Janet understand why she was vulnerable in the first place, and to stay well.

In the realm of the transpersonal, there can be complex scenarios. The last two cases illustrate admixtures of spirit release and past life therapy.

---

6. The therapeutic approach described here is that advocated by William Baldwin (1992).

Release of a Lost Soul

Barbara, my patient, had been visiting a well-known museum and wanted to look at the paintings on the first floor. There was a big central staircase with stairwells on both sides. Halfway up, she started feeling dizzy and could not proceed. Since that time a few months back, open spaces and heights triggered severe panic attacks.

> I invited Barbara to close her eyes and imagine herself back at the bottom of the stairs. She became visibly tense and I asked her to focus on the sensation of fear and go with the feeling to the very first time it happened, wherever that might be. With some surprise, Barbara reported that she was standing at the bottom of a stone pyramid with big steps leading upwards and a sheer drop on each side. She was wearing rough leather sandals and a long cotton skirt. I asked her what she was doing there. She replied that she was going to be sacrificed by the chief priest. She could see him waiting for her at the top of the pyramid, where he would cut her throat.
>
> How had she come to be chosen? This took her back to a scene in the village the night before, when the elders had singled her out and said 'It might as well be her'. She had no relatives to protect her and so she was dragged away. I asked her to go back further, to her childhood in that lifetime. She told me her name was Miria. By nature, she was a solitary child, who liked to play alone in the forest. Later, being fiercely independent, she scared away her suitors, which left her with no husband to protect her and no status in village life.
>
> As if in a trance, Miria now climbed slowly up the pyramid steps. The height made her dizzy. At the top, she was lifted on to a stone slab and the priest raised his sword. Then it was over – there was no pain and she was free. Miria floated away from the body but remained suspended in a shadowy, featureless world. I asked her to look around and tell me if she could see anyone. Looking down, Miria saw a five-year-old girl playing alone in the fields behind some houses. As she came closer, she could see that it was the child Barbara. Miria felt attracted to the little girl and so she stayed with her.
>
> From the transpersonal perspective, Miria's spirit had remained earthbound, seeking solace in the company of another solitary child. The attachment only surfaced when the museum steps triggered a resurgence of fear in Miria, which had instantly and deeply affected my patient Barbara. Once this was explained to Miria, she agreed to leave. I encouraged her to look for the light, and after a short while, she found herself moving rapidly towards it and was gone.

This case raises an interesting possibility: if, as current physics suggests, space-time is a single entity, every event that ever occurred may continue to exist in its own space-time locale. It only seems to us to be 'in the past' because we have left it behind. While the normal waking state anchors us in our contemporaneous locale, in altered states of consciousness these locales may become confluent across space-time, be they drawn from the well of one's own experience or indeed from other people's lives. It may no longer be possible to say what is 'mine' and what is 'yours'.

A Soul Bereaved

Helen, in her forties, had become suddenly aware of feeling deeply emotionally burdened. There was nothing she could identify to account for it. All she could say was that she could feel a woman's presence calling out to her in distress. Helen wanted to understand more about this voice speaking to her from within. Through hypnotic induction, I was able to make direct contact with the woman, Marianne, as she called herself, and this is her story.

> Marianne had lived several centuries ago. Her mother had died in childbirth and she had been brought up by her father who was an impoverished crofter. As a small child, she fell ill and the father, at his wit's end, left her close to death on the doorstep of a convent. The mother superior found the child there and took her in. Marianne was nursed back to health, and although deeply affected by the loss of her father, she grew to love the mother superior, who showed her great kindness. The convent became her home.
>
> When she was little more than a child, there was a civil uprising and a band of drunken militia broke into the convent. Mother superior insisted that Marianne hide herself and then went out with the other nuns to face the militia. The nuns were all raped and killed. Marianne could hear what was happening and was terrified. Later, she crept out to find bodies everywhere. Weeping, she ran into the nearby woods and there, overwhelmed with guilt at not saving her beloved mother superior, she hung herself. Immediately she found herself, in spirit, back at the convent, unable to leave the scene of the massacre. From that time on, she wandered alone in a state of shock and deeply burdened by guilt, until she found herself attracted to Helen and 'moved in'.
>
> The therapeutic task was to take this traumatised soul back to her suicide and help her complete the transition to the afterlife. As soon as she crossed over, the first person to greet her was the mother superior. Marianne wept and asked for forgiveness. The mother superior embraced her, saying, 'You have nothing to blame yourself for.' Marianne answered, 'But how can I repay all you did for me?' The mother superior replied, 'I have waited a long time for you to come and you are repaying me now by enabling me to be the first person to greet you.'
>
> Then Marianne looked round and saw her father. He had died a few years after leaving his child at the door of the convent. Still in anguish as to whether he had done the right thing, he asked her to forgive him. Finally,

Marianne's mother, who she had never known, appeared and lovingly greeted her. For the first time this family was complete and reunited.

Marianne never troubled Helen again. The therapeutic effect was profound, for it also addressed a lifelong concern of Helen's: feeling that it was dangerous to love without reservation, for fear of abandonment. In a letter some months later, Helen wrote that both she and Marianne had been released from what she called 'the trap of abandonment'.

Through witnessing Marianne's reunion, first with the mother superior and then with her parents, it was impressed on Helen that no one in Marianne's family had wished to cause hurt and rejection; on the contrary, their love for Marianne was plain to see. In the light of this experience, Helen could now recognise that her own family, imperfect though it may have been, had done its best for her.

In Conclusion

What is required for soul-centred therapy? Firstly, willingness to consider spiritual reality to be as 'real' as any aspect of life; secondly, readiness to work beyond the bounds of mundane reality; and thirdly, trust that our patients already hold the key to their own healing.

I am not advocating soul-centred therapy as a catch-all, for the individual need must always be assessed. Sometimes a person will use 'spirituality' as a defence against confronting painful emotion in the here-and-now. Other times, it is better simply to work through a problem staying firmly grounded in the affairs of daily life. However, in the examples given here, the chosen field of action has been psycho-spiritual, unconstrained by the limits of physical reality, not least birth and death. The aim is always to throw light on the complex challenges of human life, mindful that each scene in the play is essential to the working out of the greater whole. To this end, I shall hope the case studies included here furnish ample evidence of the depth and wisdom of the human soul.

References

Baldwin, W. (1992) *Spirit Releasement Therapy*. Headline Books.
Leitenberg, M. (2006) *Deaths in Wars and Conflicts in the 20th century*. (Cornell University Peace Studies Program Occasional Paper no. 29). Cornell University. Available at: http://www.clingendael.nl/sites/default/files/20060800_cdsp_occ_leitenberg.pdf (accessed 4th July 2017).
Powell, A. (2017) *The Ways of the Soul. A Psychiatrist Reflects: Essays on Life, Death and Beyond*. Muswell Hill Press.

7

Healing and the Wounded Psyche

I first became interested in the subject of healing[1] in my forties. The reasons were both personal and professional, and I had no idea at the time how my life would change.

For a number of years I had been working as a consultant psychotherapist in a large hospital, involved in teaching, supervision and seeing patients for individual and group psychotherapy. I had revered Sigmund Freud, feeling myself to be standing on the shoulders of a giant, and I was bent on helping my patients to the best of my ability. I believed that my knowledge of unconscious mental processes gave me a privileged insight into the workings of the human mind.

Psychoanalysis is aligned with the Newtonian world-view. The psychology is reductionist, mapping in detail the components of the mind and the mechanisms that govern its function, while aiming to help resolve fractious parts into a better functioning whole. The problem of where the mind actually resides or how it relates to the brain has remained largely unaddressed. Great attention has been given, however, to the complex, dynamic factors that shape the development of personality.

To begin with, the explanatory power of psychoanalysis had greatly attracted me, but over the years I began to feel uncomfortable with what I felt to be its limitations. While claiming to encompass all of the human mind, psychoanalysis as a secular theory had no place for the soul, nor showed any regard for spiritual reality. Freud was a confirmed atheist, having turned his back on the Jewish mystical tradition.

Paper prepared for conference 'Spiritual and Religious Healing: Implications for Mental Healthcare', held by the Spirituality and Psychiatry Special Interest Group at the Royal College of Psychiatrists, London, April 2010.

---

1. Often referred to as 'hands-on healing', this is really a misnomer, for many healers work without physically touching the body. For an account of research into healing that is both personal and professional, see Bengston (2010).

His investigation into the workings of the unconscious mined a rich vein, but he took the consciousness of everyday life to be the highest and best to which the human being may aspire. In fact, Freud disparaged the transcendental, feeling it to be a threat to the good name of psychoanalysis.

I was increasingly drawn to the writings of Carl Jung. Whereas Freud minutely examined the mind rather like the engine of a car, Jung's attention was focussed on the self, an inclusive vision which dared ask questions of the driver as much as looking under the bonnet. At the heart of Jung's exploration lies God, although Jung liked to use the term Imago Dei when exploring the psychology of the sacred.

Jung's readiness to see each person as sharing in a deep ocean of knowledge, the collective unconscious, attracted him to advances in quantum physics and the investigation of what Freud had scathingly dismissed – the so-called paranormal. Through his work with active imagination and the archetypes, Jung recognised that while we see through a glass darkly, we can nevertheless envision something of the greater whole from whence our individual psyches have arisen. At heart, Jung was a gnostic.[2]

To return to the existential predicament in which I found myself at the time, I knew there was more work to be done. As I had been in psychoanalysis previously, should I return to the couch for more?

In trying to understand how the mind works, psychoanalysis has proved adept at uncovering the ruses, deceptions and distortions employed by the ego to stay in the driving seat. It is good, of course, to know *about* oneself – to be cognisant of one's ego, its vulnerabilities and defences. However, I did not discover *who* I am, for analytical introspection engenders the subject–object divide. While a person as subject can learn about themselves as the object of their reflection, the object cannot be known from within, since it can never be the subject. I could see that ego psychology, having no regard for the soul, was not going to take me where I needed to go – to the spiritual essence of one's being and wherein lies the source of healing.

I decided instead to explore the esoteric tradition, which is undisguisedly centred on wholeness of being, in relation not only to individual consciousness, but also the greater transpersonal consciousness of the cosmos – thus the saying 'as above, so below'.[3]

---

2. The Greek word *gnosis* means to become conscious *of* oneself, not to be confused with rationality (cf. Latin *ratio*, to measure), which is to learn *about* oneself.
3. From the inscription on the fabled Emerald Tablet of Hermes Trismegistus: 'That which is above is like that which is below and that which is below is like

Interestingly, this axiom of ancient alchemy is now corroborated by the physics of quantum entanglement that describes a unitary energy field superordinate to the rule set of Newtonian physics. Two photons once entangled but then separated in space continue to react instantaneously to each other. Stop the integer spin of one and the other stops simultaneously. There is no time lag, not even at the speed of light. This is superluminal connection, and strong evidence for an overarching domain that transcends the limits of time and space.[4] Consequently, it is now possible to approach the whole field of paranormal research in a thoughtful and open-minded way.[5] Further, the door is opened to an understanding of healing research[6] through effects that have always been inexplicable according to classical physics.

To continue, however, with my own story, I decided to find out what the College of Healing in Malvern had to offer. Later, I attended the School of Channelling there as well. I learned a great deal from the experience of working with healers and subsequently began to include the transpersonal dimension in my work with some patients.

Healing as an energy exchange requires the healer to focus on the healee with both compassion and dispassion. The healer's mind is emptied of all thoughts except to attune to the energies of the healee, many healers asking only that 'Thy will be done'. In this way, the healer acts as a channel for an inflow of energy that finds its way to where it is needed, to relieve pain and promote tissue regeneration and repair.

There are many kinds of healing. Healers who are 'medical intuitives' visualise structural pathology rather like an X-ray and 'scan' accordingly. Other healers 'feel' the human energy field (aura) as they make passes with their hands above the body surface while giving healing and 'balancing' to the energy centres of the body, known as *chakras*.[7] Some healers work with specific imagery while others leave it to 'the powers that be'. Yet other healers clairvoyantly see spirit presences or angelic forms standing around the healee, who may identify themselves as doctors and nurses from the spirit world. Brazilian psychic surgeons, such as Jose Arigó and João de Deus, have used penknives, probes and scissors to cut into the body – apparently never with any post-operative

---

      that which is above… This is the foundation of astrology and alchemy: that the microcosm of mankind and the earth is a reflection of the macrocosm of God and the heavens'. For more on Hermetic philosophy, see Mead (2016).
4. See also *Modernity and the Beleaguered Soul*, this volume.
5. For a comprehensive account, see Radin (1997; 2006).
6. Benor (2002).
7. For a discussion of the *chakras*, see *Varieties of Love and the Near-Life Experience*, in Powell (2017).

infection. Filipino healers like Alex Orbito use their hands to 'enter' the body and extract diseased tissue.

A physician friend of mine took his wife, who had an abdominal tumour, to the Philippines and stood next to her while she was operated on. He watched the healer's hand apparently penetrate his wife's abdomen and extract a large lump of bloody tissue. When the blood was swabbed away, there was no visible trauma to the abdominal wall. At the time of the 'operation' my friend had no doubt of the reality of his perception. Afterwards, cognitive dissonance set in and made him question whether he had imagined what he thought he had seen. At any rate, his wife got better.

These procedures have been examined and emphatically pronounced fraudulent by James Randi, magician and sceptic, who spearheads a campaign to discredit psychic and spiritual healers. Can one believe one's eyes? The art of misdirection is subtle. That is why rigorous empirical research is so important.[8]

I can relate my own experience of psychic surgery when I consulted Stephen Turoff, who 'brings through' a deceased Viennese physician called Dr Kahn. Stephen is a cheery ex-plumber who, as a young man, suddenly fell into trance. When he came round, he was told that a stranger had seemingly spoken through him in a voice with a foreign accent, requesting permission to use Stephen as a healer and spirit surgeon. Stephen agreed, on condition that he would not have to see any blood, as he was rather squeamish.

I went to see Turoff in 1993, since I had a deteriorating heart valve. I was in no hurry for cardiac surgery, so meantime I was exploring anything that might help. When I met 'Dr Kahn', I really did seem to be conversing with a twinkling eyed, elderly and rather old-fashioned physician with a strong foreign accent. I began to give my medical history but Dr Kahn did not seem much interested. He told me to take my shirt off, thrust me down on the couch and began 'operating' on me. It was an extraordinary experience. He worked at high speed, like a video in fast forward, scratching at my sternum with nail scissors and repeatedly extracting, so it seemed, something from my chest. Each time he appeared to throw it in the direction of the metal waste bin where it landed with a clinking sound. Dr Kahn's concentration was intense and the whole thing lasted only a few minutes. It ended with his pressing his hand on my chest for about 30 seconds, as if to stem the flow of blood. Afterwards there was a red mark, which faded over a few days.

---

8. For a scholarly meta-analysis of non-contact healing, see Roe et al. (2015).

When Stephen Turoff had left the room, I got up and looked in the waste paper bin. It was empty except for some cotton wool swabs. Later, reading a biography of Turoff, I found out that in order to spare Turoff the sight of blood or gore, Dr Kahn had promised to dematerialise any physical matter he extracted. I told a physicist friend about this, who pointed out that if matter could indeed be dematerialised just like that, it would create a vacuum. As with lightning, but on a micro scale, the collapse of the vacuum would be certain to be audible.

At my follow-up appointment, I decided to ask Dr Kahn whether my heart valve problem might be attributable to karma – not impossible if one holds that mind and matter arise from the same source. Dr Kahn peered at me through his glasses, and then burst out laughing, saying 'Sometimes a cigar is only a cigar!' This was an extraordinary reply, one that I understood perfectly, although it was the last thing I expected to hear from an ex-plumber. Freud did not hesitate to analyse his patients' oral fixations but concerning his own habit of cigar smoking (which eventually resulted in cancer of the jaw) he would only say, 'Sometimes a cigar is only a cigar!'

I had in mind to ask about my prognosis but was feeling rather anxious. Dr Kahn looked at me intently and said, 'You know, I can see what the future holds for you'. My anxiety level soared. He added, 'You don't need to worry. You have many years ahead'. I walked out feeling like a man reprieved and so far he has been proven right.

When I went back to my cardiologist for my next echocardiogram, he said, 'This is very surprising. Your measurements have all improved!' They remained stable for the next two years, when suddenly I became acutely ill and my valve had to be replaced. That was over 20 years ago.

Healing is a particularly interesting phenomenon because it spans the worlds of material realism and the metaphysical. Medically speaking, the use of the term is confined to natural repair – fibroblasts migrate to sites of tissue injury and form scar tissue, bony fractures unite due to a proliferation of osteoblasts and so on. Something is at work orchestrating tissue repair. We talk about mechanisms like chemotaxis, yet we do not really know what organising forces are at work. Even so, forces there must be, for we see the evidence in healers' ability to induce the early germination of seeds,[9] to waken anaesthetised mice[10] and to accelerate wound healing.[11] 'Distance healing' does not follow the usual laws of physics, for its effects are independent

---
9. Grad (1965); Saklani (1998).
10. Watkins & Watkins (1971).
11. Grad et al. (1961).

of the proximity of the healer,[12] while studies such as those on the effect of retroactive prayer[13] and on presentiment[14,15] appear to violate the principle of linear time.

Healing, then, takes us beyond the mundane world to worlds unseen, a universe of energy and interconnectedness that is way outside the physicalist Newtonian world-view. While we might have expected to confine healing to the re-alignment of natural but subtle energies, now that the laws of space and time are breached, birth and death no longer hold the same finite meaning. Instead, they might be better conceived of as discontinuous phase transitions.

According to the Buddhist tradition, there is no enduring soul that survives death. However, my researches, including many survivor reports of the near-death experience, have persuaded me of the survival of the soul – not one that rests on its laurels, but one that constantly strives to move forward and to grow in understanding and wisdom. Those inclined towards this view will appreciate the contributions of David Fontana,[16] who founded the Transpersonal Section of the British Psychological Society.

How much can a person do in one short lifespan? It seems likely to me that we go through many lifetimes, very possibly in different locales of space-time, before approaching anything like the wisdom of the spiritual masters. If this mundane life is a classroom for the soul, then the law of karma, which states that cause invariably leads to effect (becoming in turn the next cause), provides a perfect psycho-spiritual blueprint for the progress of humanity. Moreover, if indeed we are participants in a spiritual cosmos,[17] it makes sense that consciousness needs to find expression in sentient species, in which case the human drama is no mere sideshow in the great scheme of things. Human life, as with all of life arising in the universe, is the means by which the universe can become conscious of itself.[18]

There are at least three good reasons for thinking it is no accident that conscious beings like us exist in such a universe. Firstly, thanks to quantum field theory, we no longer think of the universe as a void populated with eruptions of gas and large lumps of rock. Instead, the

---

12. See Byrd (1988); Harris et al. (1999).
13. Leibovici (2001).
14. Radin (1997).
15. For a peer-reviewed and methodologically rigorous trial, see Bem (2011).
16. Fontana (2005).
17. For an illuminating study of the evolutionary cosmos, see Swimme & Tucker (2011).
18. This presumably is the purpose of the subject–object divide on a grand scale.

evidence points to an unseen but apparently limitless flux of energy, constantly giving birth to physical matter with the collapse of the wave function and dissolving back into itself according to the law of entropy. The physicist Amit Goswami[19] describes this reciprocity as a tangled hierarchy, in which consciousness brings about the collapse of the wave and the collapse of the wave brings about consciousness, rather as in Maurits Escher's famous picture *Drawing Hands*.[20]

A second reason concerns the holographic nature of the universe. Michael Talbot[21] has described how the converging insights of two great scientists of our time led to this revolutionary concept. Karl Pribram, the neurophysiologist, had been searching for a topographical basis to memory in the brain but could not identify any physical localisation of function. When he learned about the new science of holograms, he developed the theory that memory is stored holographically by means of arrays of neurons producing electrical interference patterns in waveform, known as Fourier transforms.[22] The visual cortex was found to work in the same way. Pribram was pondering the implications of this finding – that everything we perceive that looks real and solid might simply be holographic projections – when he came across the work of the quantum physicist David Bohm.

Bohm had concluded that the whole physical universe is itself a holographic projection, being the *explicate* order of an invisible, deeper *implicate* order, in the same way that when a laser beam strikes a photographic plate on which is embedded an interference pattern, it will generate a three-dimensional image. Bohm wrote:

> 'Ultimately, the entire universe (with all its particles, including those constituting human beings, their laboratories, observing instruments, etc.) has to be understood as a single undivided whole, in which analysis into separately and independently existent parts has no fundamental status'.[23]

Talbot summarises it like this: 'Our brains mathematically construct objective reality by interpreting frequencies that are ultimately projections from another dimension, a deeper order of existence that is beyond both time and space: the brain is a hologram enfolded in a

---

19. Goswami (1993).
20. A lithograph printed in 1948 depicting a sheet of paper out of which, from wrists that remain flat on the page, two hands rise, facing each other and in the paradoxical act of drawing one another into existence.
21. Talbot (1991).
22. See Pribram (1977).
23. Bohm (1980: 74).

holographic universe'.[24] Consciousness is therefore intrinsic to the universe as we know it.

A third reason for thinking we are deeply implicated in the life of the universe is to give credence to intuition. The great 17th-century scientist and mystic Blaise Pascal wrote: 'the heart has its reasons of which reason knows nothing'.[25] Isaac Newton, born in the same century, is said to have described his method as, firstly, mystical intuition into implicate truth; secondly, mathematical intellection, to prove, express or explicate the implicate understanding; and thirdly, experimentation, in order to demonstrate and verify the proof.[26] Closer to our time, the brilliant polymath Henri Poincaré was to write that it is through science that we prove, but through intuition that we discover.

How can this be so? The science of holographic cosmology may hold the key.[27] Since in a hologram the part contains the whole, instead of discounting the subjective, we can try looking within ourselves for the answer. Within the implicate order, to use Bohm's term, we *are* one with all that is.

Nonetheless, we perceive ourselves in the phenomenal world as separate entities. This is the domain of the ego, to which we humans are indebted for our evolution as a species. Yet the ego, too, is only a function of the mind, and the mind is not really a thing at all – it is a process. Even when we talk about the physical brain as a thing, from the holographic perspective it, too, is merely an energetic process, fashioned into something solid by our special sense organs. Nothing has any objective reality or solidity beyond the consciousness that is ultimately what we are. From this perspective, birth, life, illness and death can be likened to ripples in the interference pattern of the implicate order.

My early acquaintance with healing was focussed on the body, but as a psychotherapist, my interest soon centred on how the mind might find healing, a path that led me to explore soul-centred therapy. I have written elsewhere about its clinical application,[28] but here I will take up the broader question of woundedness as set against the backdrop of a 'living' universe and the vast intelligence that it expresses.

Why cannot human beings simply live in Paradise? Why did Adam and Eve have to be exiled from the Garden of Eden? This profound

---

24. Talbot (1991: 54).
25. Trotter (2005: 277).
26. Newton is also widely quoted as having said, in his old age, that truth is the offspring of silence and unbroken meditation.
27. For an illuminating and comprehensive review, see Currivan (2017).
28. *Soul-Centred Psychotherapy*, this volume.

myth describes the fate of every human infant, for there is no childhood without trauma, frustration, pain, rejection and loss.

In the first place, the human drama being played out so tenaciously can be seen as supporting the further evolution of consciousness. We each make our personal contribution as we learn how to withstand the demands of the ego and to align ourselves with the values of the soul all the greater when we do so collectively, in harness with a universe moving in the same direction.[29]

Secondly, while the soul brings unconditional love to the ego, the ego brings experience of life to the soul. If we could stay in a perpetual comfort zone, we would learn nothing. Very possibly this is why the soul is driven to incarnate in the first place.

The ego is instrumental in the construction of the personality, a complex amalgam born out of the needs and desires of the child learning to grow and survive in a competitive and unpredictable world. Yet, ironically, the ego is the servant of spiritual growth, for in its ambition to conquer all, it must eventually face losing all. The wounds to the ego are countless – fear of loss of status, of material possessions, of being loved and finally, of death are all consequences of its separative mentality.

The soul, in contrast, unfolds from the implicate order to manifest in each human being. Furthermore, the incarnated soul does not love for reasons of need, like the ego. On the contrary, it is the radiation of sheer, unconditional love – which knows the final outcome to be good. Where, how and when, we cannot say, but as Mother Julian of Norwich proclaimed 700 years ago, '…all will be well and all manner of things will be well'.[30]

The soul is unperturbed by death, since it is perfectly at ease with the transience of human life. However, in cohabiting with the ego for the purposes of gaining experience, the soul must share in the ego's experience of pain, rejection and abuse. This is the great test of a person's humanity, as found in the words of Jesus, '…but I tell you, love your enemies and pray for those who persecute you'.[31] Helping us to go on loving in the face of being wounded is the soul's agenda. It calls for forgiveness where the impulse of the ego is to retaliate. Retaliation constricts the heart but forgiveness expands it. Forgiveness is not confined to forgiving others, for when we see we have hurt others we are faced with finding forgiveness for ourselves too. Yet when we understand that ultimately humanity is one, compassion for others and for oneself is the one and same thing.

---

29. See *Why Must We Suffer? A Psychiatrist Reflects*, this volume.
30. Backhouse (1987: 56).
31. Matthew 5:44. *The Holy Bible*, NIV.

Most importantly, there need be no incongruity between human psychology and the spiritual agenda. As protagonists in the theatre of life, we humans live through a thousand scenes, each one to be experienced deeply, authentically and in the most personal way. The lines are written and yet the script is open to endless improvisation. We do not have to follow the plot – there is freedom of action. Nevertheless, if we do not accomplish what we came to discover and do, the soul will be the poorer for it.

This is where I want to come back to healing, bestowed by the soul as an act of unconditional love. With the help of the healer, the healee is brought into alignment with their own wholeness of being. Where there is dis-ease and dis-unity, coherency is restored to mind and body, giving the best chance for recovery of health. Yet healing is also important where bodily decline is inevitable. Here, the aim is to minimise physical and emotional stress and to bring peace and comfort. The Greek root of the word for therapy is *therapeuein*, which does not just mean to treat; it means to serve, to care for and to heal.

Love is a word largely avoided in the lexicon of psychiatry and psychotherapy, understandably perhaps, given its association with the possessive and destructive potential of the ego. Nevertheless, we should not hesitate to bring the soul into the consulting room, for whether the doctor is a surgeon, physician or psychiatrist, the presence of unconditional love will enhance every kind of treatment. What is broken will be helped to mend, what is wounded will be helped to heal. We are born whole, we become disunited and we spend our lives searching for that sense of wholeness we once knew. Yet we cannot return to where we began, nor is it intended we should. Instead, as T.S. Eliot writes, it is 'to arrive at the place we started and know the place for the first time'.[32] That is the birth of a new consciousness, and the start of a new journey.

References

Backhouse, H. (ed.) (1987) *Julian of Norwich: Revelations of Divine Love*. Hodder & Stoughton.
Bem, D. (2011) Feeling the future: experimental evidence for anomalous retroactive influence on cognition and affect. *Journal of Personality and Social Psychology*, 100, 407–425.
Bengston, W. (2010) *The Energy Cure: Unraveling the Mystery of Hands-On Healing*. Sounds True.
Benor, D. (2002) *Healing Research*, vol. 1, Spiritual Healing: Scientific Validation of a Healing Revolution. Vision Publications.

---

32. Elliot (1999).

Bohm, D. (1980) *Wholeness and the Implicate Order*. Routledge.
Byrd, R. (1988) Positive therapeutic effects of intercessory prayer in a coronary care population. *Southern Medical Journal*, 81, 826–829.
Currivan, J. (2017) *The Cosmic Hologram*. Inner Traditions.
Elliot, T.S. (1999) Little Gidding. In *Four Quartets*. Faber & Faber.
Fontana, D. (2005) *Is There An Afterlife?* O Books.
Goswami, A. (1993) *The Self-Aware Universe*. Tarcher/Putnam.
Grad, B., Cadoret, R, & Paul, G. (1961) The influence of an unorthodox method of treatment on wound healing in mice. *International Journal of Parapsychology*, 3, 5–24.
Grad, B. (1965) Some biological effects of the 'laying on of hands': a review of experiments with animals and plants. *Journal of the American Society for Psychical Research*, 59, 95–127.
Harris, W., Gowda, M., Kolb, J.W., et al. (1999) A randomized controlled trial of the effects of remote intercessory prayer on outcomes in patients admitted to the coronary care unit. *Annals of Internal Medicine*, 159, 2273–2278.
Leibovici, L. (2001) Effects of remote, retroactive intercessory prayer on outcomes in patients with bloodstream infection: randomised controlled trial. *BMJ*, 323, 1450–1451.
Mead, G.R.S. (2016) *The Corpus Hermeticum: Initiation Into Hermetics. The Hermetica of Hermes Trismegistus*. Create Space Independent Publishing Platform.
Powell, A. (2017) *The Ways of the Soul. A Psychiatrist Reflects: Essays on Life, Death and Beyond*. Muswell Hill Press.
Pribram, K. (1971) *Languages of the Brain*. Brandon House.
Radin, D. (1997) *The Conscious Universe*. HarperCollins.
Radin, D. (2006) *Entangled Minds*. Paraview Pocket Books.
Roe, C., Sonnex, C., & Roxburgh, E. (2015) Two meta-analyses of non-contact healing studies. *Explore*, 11, 11–23.
Saklani, A. (1988) Psi-ability in shamans of Garhwal Himalaya: preliminary tests. *Journal of the Society for Psychical Research*, 55, 60–70.
Swimme, B. & Tucker, M. (2011) *Journey of the Universe*. Yale University Press.
Talbot, M. (1991) *The Holographic Universe*. HarperCollins.
Trotter, W.F. (transl.) (2005) *Blaise Pascal: Pensées (Thoughts)*. Section IV: 'Of the Means of Belief'. Digireads.com.
Watkins, G. & Watkins, A. (1971) Possible PK influences on the resuscitation of anesthetized mice. *Journal of Parapsychology,* 35(4), 257–272.

8

Open Heart, Open Mind: Conversing with the Soul

On the subject of conversing with the soul, I would like to begin by discussing empathy, which opens the way for souls to meet. Empathy is not to be confused with projection, in which a person has unwittingly confused what they are feeling with what they suppose the other to be feeling. Empathy is the capacity to put oneself in the shoes of the other and to see, as far as it is possible, the world through someone else's eyes.

The capacity for empathy develops in the first year of life. Functional magnetic resonance imaging (fMRI)[1] has shown that from babyhood onwards, mirror neurons in the pre-frontal cortex and somatosensory areas of the child's brain are activated by mother–child interactions, enabling an imaginative comprehension of the inner world of the other.[2]

Perhaps surprisingly, many psychopaths have the capacity for empathy. A torturer knows that a person under interrogation may bravely face his own death but will capitulate if the threat is made to murder the prisoner's family. This kind of coercion requires empathic identification with the prisoner. However, the psychopath is not in touch with what it means to love. Such 'intellectual empathy' can be a dangerous weapon when used in the service of manipulation.

For the majority of us who are moved both by our conscience and by our feelings, empathy is the prerequisite of love in its most unselfish form – compassion. The human race is a young species in planetary time, certainly less than 2 million years old, and only during the past

---

Paper prepared for conference 'Physicians of the Soul: Between Psychotherapy and Spirituality', Trinity College, University of Oxford, September 2011.

1. Functional magnetic resonance imaging enables brain mapping by measuring changes in blood flow when areas of the brain are activated.
2. Keysers et al. (2010).

200,000 years has complex social life with speech and symbolisation developed. Compassion for kith and kin doubtless flourished in tribal communities, bent on sheer survival and protective of the social group. Yet the ethos of having compassion for one's enemies is very recent when set against the timeline of humanity and is far from universal, as today's climate of terrorist atrocities bears witness.

Compassion is, nevertheless, found at the heart of all the major faith traditions. In the field of medicine, too, it has always been indispensable to good medical practice, which does not distinguish between friend and foe. Yet from psychoanalysis through to the plethora of psychological treatments that have flourished since, there has been far greater interest in empathy than compassion. Why should this be so?

My impression is that offering love, albeit of the compassionate variety, is felt by most mental health professionals, including psychotherapists, to overstep the bounds of propriety. We do not speak of loving our patients or even having love for our patients for fear that this will be regarded as an inappropriate emotion, too personal in nature and one that may lead to unprofessional intimacy. Instead, we suspend judgement, demonstrate concern, pay attention, show interest and do a good deal of 'containing'.

The aim is to enable our patients to find a greater degree of self-understanding and so help them live healthier and happier lives. Yet there are dangers too. Firstly, the therapist may hold a view about what is to be regarded as normal that can render an anxious or depressed person captive to the therapist's ambitions for them. Secondly, employing a favoured therapeutic approach may say more about the therapist's personal interest and preference than what is best for the patient. Last but not least, if the therapy is carried out mind-to-mind and the heart is unattended, the essence of the person seeking help remains untouched.[3] The therapist will never truly have 'met' their patient and the patient will know it and feel it. No technique alone can bring about healing; a relationship is needed.

Despite the best efforts of clinicians, we are dealing these days with an extraordinary epidemic of mental anguish and we have to question why this should be so. Some psychiatrists[4] have argued that the real sickness lies not in the patient but in society itself, and that medicalising or psychologising emotional distress, however well intentioned, is a symptom of the same illness.

---

3. As adjudged by the apostle Paul, 'If I speak in the tongues of men or of angels, but do not have love, I am only a resounding gong or a clanging cymbal'. 1 Corinthians 13. *The Holy Bible*, NIV.
4. Most famously, Thomas Szasz. See Szasz (1961).

I do not refer here to the 2% or so of the population living with severe mental illness, namely bipolar disorder and schizophrenia, but the current epidemic of depression, with over 60 million prescriptions for antidepressants in the UK in 2015 and still rising.[5] Psychological treatments are similarly being rolled out nationwide.[6] Yet the root cause of so much depression is not being examined, perhaps because it puts a question mark against our whole way of life. My concern is with just this – a secular, consumerist world that oftentimes seems to 'know the price of everything and the value of nothing',[7] and in which symptoms of the soul in anguish are taken to be a sign of illness.

Should this matter be the subject of psychological or spiritual enquiry – or both? The therapist who presses their own spiritual viewpoint on their patient would be insensitive at best and abusive at worst. Yet a treatment that focuses only on the psychological level when the soul is crying out to be heard can be compared with moving furniture around when the house is falling down!

I began by introducing the subject of empathy, thence to compassion, and now I have moved on to the soul, the seat of compassion. Here I should briefly explain how I am using the word soul in the hope that I may shed some light on why love has become split off from therapy – much to be regretted, since unconditional love is the wellspring of healing.

By no means does everyone believe in the eternal nature of the soul. Nevertheless, it is possible to affirm that there is, in each of us, an essence that appears to be undeterred by the trauma and suffering that attends life, that manifests as love even in the most unlikely circumstances and, most importantly, that loves without counting the cost. This kind of love is not based on physical desire, nor does it seek security. There is only the wish for the welfare and happiness of oneself and others.

Such is the nature of soul love. Every human is capable of it, although sadly, many people do not realise they have it in them. The ego cannot know about this because its concern is always with itself. However, the soul is well aware that we are all, without exception, in the same boat, and that regardless of our differences we share the same hopes, fears and dreams, even unto death. In this sense, we are one, and to hurt the other is only to hurt the self. This is the basis of the golden

---

5. NHS Digital (2016).
6. In 2008, a nationwide programme called Improving Access to Psychological Therapies (IAPT) was set up by NHS England, offering short-term counselling and cognitive–behavioural therapy for adults.
7. A notable turn of phrase by Oscar Wilde (from *Lady Windermere's Fan*).

rule, the cornerstone of the great faith traditions: 'Do not do to others as you would not have them do to you', also known more simply as 'Love your neighbour as yourself'.

I would like briefly to turn to science in support of the transpersonal psychology I want to introduce here, bearing in mind that human faculties allow us only a small glimpse of a reality far greater than our senses allow.[8]

With the caveat that each person – myself included – seeks out, consciously or otherwise, the evidence that will support their preferred point of view, I have come to the conclusion that consciousness is not derivative but primary. Since consciousness cannot be put under the microscope, it has, for the purposes of science, remained the elephant in the room. Indirectly, however, and with the help of quantum modelling, we have been able to determine some of its characteristics – most importantly, that consciousness is non-local and extends throughout and beyond space-time. Put differently, we might say that information is seeded throughout the cosmos, and since the cosmos appears to be structured holographically, 'God' is everywhere and in everything, including all of us.[9]

I mention this to emphasise that when speaking of the metaphysical soul, I am viewing the whole cosmos as a living organism which finds expression in both material form and consciousness – two sides of the same coin.[10] It seems to me that the sterile debate of monism versus dualism arises because this perspective is missing.

However small we human beings may be in the cosmic scale of things, we nevertheless are blessed with an awareness of the greater whole. It also makes sense to me that the evolution of consciousness enables us to play our part in helping God to know more of *that which is God*. While staying clear of complicated theological arguments, I am arguing for an evolutionary process at work within our dimension of space-time (perhaps the whole point of such dimensions). Therein lies our privilege and responsibility to advance the consciousness of humankind for reasons that serve both humanity and divinity.

Finally, if we may infer from the mathematics of the Mandelbrot set that our universe is most likely structured holographically, no matter

---

8. The transpersonal has been defined as 'experiences in which the sense of identity or self extends beyond (*trans*) the individual or personal to encompass wider aspects of humankind, life, psyche or cosmos'. Walsh & Vaughan (1993: 203).
9. Regardless of whether the existence of God is rejected or affirmed, as an archetype the Imago Dei is always present in the collective unconscious.
10. The subject is dealt with in more depth in *Beyond Space and Time – The Unbounded Psyche*, in Powell (2017).

how dark the glass through which we see, our human capacity for love is thereby a reflection of the greater design.

What might such a transpersonal perspective mean for psychotherapeutic work in mental healthcare?[11] How and when is it right to explore matters of spirituality and/or religion with one's patient?[12] This is not something about which to be prescriptive. Nonetheless, there are times in the therapeutic encounter when the 'big questions' arise. Why am I here? Where did I come from? What is the point of life? Why must I suffer? What happens when I die? Is there a God? Will I be judged? We know that patients are highly sensitive to both the interests and prejudices of their therapists, and the therapist who is uncomfortable with these deep questions of the soul will subtly discourage them from finding expression. On the other hand, if the therapist is open to them, especially at times of crisis, they may well be voiced.

I might have called these the big existential questions, for indeed they are. Nevertheless, I prefer to call them spiritual questions because the existential thesis argues for the primacy of human reality, whereas the transpersonal perspective holds that human reality is nested within a greater consciousness. Whether my personal identity endures or what form it may take is open to question, but either way, I envisage a participative cosmos in which I am in relation to the greater whole – the *anima mundi* (world soul) and beyond that, the *anima universale*.

Some psychiatrists would argue that to be overly concerned with such daunting questions is suggestive of a depressive disorder that would be better relieved by pharmaceutical or psychological means. Many psychoanalysts, too, feel that these preoccupations naturally fade into the background when the goals of analysis – finding fulfilment in work, love and recreation – are achieved. However, there is another stratum to the reluctance of psychoanalysis to engage with spirituality. Sigmund Freud saw death as the inevitable outcome of the opposing instincts: Eros, the life instinct, and the death instinct (later called Thanatos), with an eventual outcome so fearful to the ego that it turns defensively to religion for comfort.

It is unfortunate that when Freud did refer to the soul (German: *Seele*) even in its secular rather than sacred meaning, it was translated by James Strachey[13] as 'mental apparatus'. At any rate, there is a dearth of psychoanalytic literature on the spirituality of life and death. The writings

---

11. The etymology of psychotherapy is from the Greek, *psyche*, meaning soul and *therapeia*, meaning curing/healing.
12. See *Whither the Soul of Psychiatry?*, this volume, for broad definitions of spirituality and religion.
13. James Strachey, translator of *The Complete Psychological Works of Sigmund Freud*.

of Frank Malone,[14] Nathan Field[15] and Alistair Ross[16] are exceptions. To this day, many psychoanalysts avoid the spiritual dimension, or feel obliged to interpret it in relation to infantile phantasy.

In contrast to Freud, Carl Jung was deeply concerned with the soul, the archetype that subsumes the animus and anima, and second only to the supreme archetype of the Self. Jung asserted that the death instinct can be met without fear and that as the wheel of life turns, we can be reconciled to death within an overarching spirituality of endless renewal.[17]

The spiritual focus was given further prominence by Roberto Assagioli,[18] a psychoanalyst deeply influenced by Jung, who founded psychosynthesis more than 50 years ago. Since that time, transpersonal psychology has fostered a range of therapeutic approaches, some with an explicit interest in altered states of consciousness and some that engage specifically with worlds unseen, often referred to as the spirit world by shamans and by spiritualist and Pentecostal churches.

Soul-centred therapies include spiritual healing, spirit release, past life regression, between-lives therapy and soul retrieval. These therapies take the practitioner and/or client into realms that are quite extraordinary when set against the consensus reality our modern society takes for normal.

I have given a range of clinical illustrations elsewhere[19] and here I shall only make a broad point. Most psychiatrists would account for what is reported in such transpersonal therapies as an elaboration of phantasy. However, this is not phantasy as we normally take it to be, for the experiences that patients describe have a striking verisimilitude to them. Unexpected narratives unfold and 'journeys' are undertaken that are vivid in every detail. Psychiatrists generally are uncomfortable with this kind of thing because so much of psychiatry relies on consensus reality for the assessment of mental health.[20] Even so, for the

---

14. Malone (2005).
15. Field (2005).
16. Ross (2010).
17. Jung writes: 'The sun, rising triumphant, tears himself from the enveloping womb of the sea, and leaving behind him the noonday zenith and all its glorious works, sinks down again into the maternal depths, into all-enfolding and all-regenerating night... And having reached the noonday heights, [Man] must sacrifice his love for his own achievement, for he may not loiter. The sun, too, sacrifices its greatest strength in order to hasten onward to the fruits of autumn, which are the seeds of rebirth'. Jung (1956: 355–356).
18. Assagioli (1975).
19. In *Soul-Centred Psychotherapy*, this volume.
20. 'Reality testing' in psychiatry involves making a judgement as to whether a

curious few there is no bar, since according to quantum mechanics, everything is possible, however improbable!

In this paper, however, I am not so much concerned with altered states of consciousness as with how we may explore the big questions simply conversing soul-to-soul. Thankfully, in such a dialogue we do not need to provide answers and neither do we need to confide our own spiritual quest. What matters is that we join empathically with our patients, taking their soul-searching as legitimate, important and to be valued.

My approach is to deepen, or take a step further, what a patient may begin by saying. For instance, if we are talking about suicide, I will ask whether the person believes it to be the absolute end. Often, the reply is 'not sure', in which case I may say, 'If there *were* to be a life beyond, how would you imagine it to be?' This can turn out to be very fruitful, addressing fear of judgement, the wish to have made amends before it is too late and discovering that what needs to die is not the body but an old way of life.

Where a person has suffered bereavement, it can help to encourage dialogue with departed loved ones. Their presence is often felt as very real. By guiding the person into a conversation, e.g. 'What do you need to ask/tell so-and-so?' followed by 'Now listen to what he/she needs to say to you' (a dialogue that can go back and forth a number of times), important unfinished business can be completed. Very often, what transpires is the need to make peace, express love and find acceptance.[21]

Problems that seem insoluble can be approached by setting aside the rational mind and asking the soul directly. One way is to ask the person to close their eyes, 'go within' and see if they can let their heart find the words (a person will often touch their chest). What would the heart say if it could speak? This is not to abandon discernment, but to correct an imbalance when the head has outrun the heart.[22]

Forgiveness is another important issue. Compassion is the essence of forgiveness, since compassion recognises that we are all flawed and that everyone is here to learn from their mistakes. The ego may not be able to forgive, since it habitually recoils when hurt, or else goes on the attack. Nevertheless, I have yet to find someone who does not wish that forgiveness might be possible one day. In this way, the seed of forgiveness is planted, although we cannot know when it will bear fruit. The

---

patient's thinking/perception is broadly consonant with consensus reality. Typically, reality testing is impaired in psychosis.
21. Powell & MacKenna (2009).
22. See also *Helping Patients Tell Their Story: Narratives of Body, Mind and Soul*, this volume.

soul rejoices, however, because it knows that in forgiveness lies healing, the soul's greatest desire, and with healing comes peace.[23]

The key to all this is that no matter how deeply the ego may be wounded, the soul, knowing only love, is unharmed. The soul may have been denied expression, but the therapist who is moved by compassion will invariably find it and help it to speak. Thinking of the soul's inestimable value, I am reminded of Dietrich Bonhoeffer, the German theologian incarcerated by the Gestapo, who turned to his interrogator when he was being tortured and said, 'You can take everything away from me but my soul'. Since, as I understand it, we do not *have* souls but *are* souls, there was ultimately nothing the Gestapo *could* take away. Preparing for his execution, Bonhoeffer quietly remarked to his fellow prisoner, 'This is the end – for me the beginning of life'.[24]

In conclusion, my wish has been to help people who have felt shattered by the travails of life to become aware of their essential soul nature, which survives all, and not just survives, but inexhaustibly loves. It is not a matter of trying to impress on someone that they *should* love, forgive or be reconciled – the ego will soon put paid to that. Yet when the soul is touched, the way opens to healing. Psychotherapy for the personality is important; a person will be all the better for knowing more about themselves. Yet when we converse with the soul, we experience our true nature, what I believe to be our divinity. Once we are shown what the best in us can be, we can set about becoming that person – no matter that it takes a lifetime.

I would like to end by returning to the notion that every person has it in them to be physician of the soul, a physician whose *therapeia* is to call the soul to action. Left to the ego, human society would remain forever rivalrous, exploitative and ignorant of the soul's greatest wish for humanity – that we have it in us to love each other as ourselves. Such a thing is only possible when, mindful of the golden rule, I see you in me and you see me in you. Then, in place of judgement, we experience empathy and the window to the soul is open.

The soul love we know as compassion has huge evolutionary significance. If humankind can begin to live in harmony with all people and with the diverse life forms on this planet, and to treat Earth with the respect she deserves, and if we learn to use science not in the service of the mind but in the service of the heart, we shall have earned ourselves a future for humanity.

---

23. As discussed in *Healing and the Wounded Psyche*, this volume.
24. Bonhoeffer (1959: 181).

References

Assagioli, R. (1975) *Psychosynthesis: A Collection of Basic Writings. A Manual of Principles and Techniques.* Turnstone Press.
Bonhoeffer, D. (1959) *Letters and Papers from Prison.* Fontana.
Field, N. (2005) *Ten Lectures on Psychotherapy and Spirituality.* Karnac Books.
Jung, C.G. (1912) The dual mother. Reprinted [1956] in *C.G. Jung: The Collected Works*, vol. 5, Symbols of Transformation (eds H. Read, M. Fordham & G. Adler). Routledge and Kegan Paul.
Keysers, C., Kaas, J. & Gazzola, V. (2010) Somatosensation in social cognition. *Nature Reviews Neuroscience*, 11, 417–428.
Malone, F. (2005) *Psychoanalysis and the Sacred.* Wyndham Hall.
NHS Digital (2016) Prescriptions dispensed in the community. Statistics for England 2005-2015. Available at http://www.hscic.gov.uk/pubs/presdisp0515 (accessed 7 July 2017).
Powell, A. & MacKenna, C. (2009) Psychotherapy. In *Spirituality and Psychiatry* (eds C.C.H. Cook, A. Powell & A. Sims). RCPsych Publications.
Powell, A. (2017) *The Ways of the Soul. A Psychiatrist Reflects: Essays on Life, Death and Beyond.* Muswell Hill Press.
Ross, A. (2010) 'Sacred Psychoanalysis': An Interpretation of the Emergence and Engagement of Religion and Spirituality in Contemporary Psychoanalysis (PhD thesis). University of Birmingham.
Szasz, T. (1961) *The Myth of Mental Illness.* HarperCollins.
Walsh, R. & Vaughan, F. (1993) On transpersonal definitions. *Journal of Transpersonal Psychology*, 25, 199–207.

9

Recovery and Well-Being: The Search for the Soul

Mental health is nourished by our capacity for love.[1] It is well recognised that we cannot wholeheartedly love others, or love life, unless we feel love for ourselves. Yet what or who is this self that each of us feels we live with as our constant companion through life?

The everyday self is shaped from infancy by all that we experience – from the baby's first feed to the parenting received, the child's peer group and on to the wider social influences. If we are fortunate to be well loved, the self that develops will keep us on track while we navigate our way through life. Finely tuned and complex in nature, this self is the crowning achievement of the ego, to which humankind is indebted for its evolutionary success as a sentient species.

Even so, life has a way of finding a person's Achilles' heel, revealing the ego to be fearful of losing what it has worked to achieve, be it fear of financial loss, the good opinion of others or the failure of personal relationships. When a person's world collapses, whether outwardly or inwardly, the existential crisis can be swift and sudden.

At such times of anguish, there is, nevertheless, a place of calm deep within we know as the soul. To use a metaphor close to home, if the ego can be likened to a gifted but wayward child, the soul stands by with the unfailing and unconditional love of a parent. Unlike the

---

Paper prepared for conference 'Spirituality, Recovery and Well-being', Heythrop College, London, March 2012.

---

1. The World Health Organization states: 'Mental health is defined as a state of well-being in which every individual realises his or her own potential, can cope with the normal stresses of life, can work productively and fruitfully, and is able to make a contribution to her or his community.' World Health Organization (2014).

turbulent emotions of the ego, the soul is constant, desiring always to bring about harmony and wholeness of being.

Wholeness arises when we are in loving relation with both self and the world. Then we discover, as Carl Rogers observed, that 'what is most personal is most general'.[2] We learn that happiness is not, as the ego would have us believe, measured by worldly success, but by keeping faith with the values of the soul.

Rather than relying on social norms as a measure of recovery from breakdown, it is important to explore how a person may align themselves with this deeper self. The mental health professional can play a crucial part in encouraging a person who has suffered breakdown to gain the confidence to live 'soulfully' – albeit in a largely intolerant and ego-driven society – by helping validate and affirm the new journey that has begun.

What is Mental Illness?

While the psychiatrist looks for symptom clusters that may suggest what treatment to provide, and despite a deluge of competing theories, mostly we still do not really know what is going on. Mental illness is an umbrella term, a mélange of wide-ranging disorders of emotion and sometimes cognition too, and although it suits to ignore the fact, a fundamental problem for psychiatry remains: consciousness and all that lies therein cannot be explained by the brain.[3] As Hamlet asserts: 'There are more things in heaven and earth, Horatio, than are dreamt of in your philosophy',[4] a salutary reminder not to fall into the delusion that neuroscience can tell us what it feels like to be a living human being. Nor can science explain how something non-material such as the mind can arise from something material such as the brain.

Psychiatry casts its diagnostic net over aspects of human thought, feeling and conduct that lie on the outer reaches of the bell-shaped normal distribution curve. Since psychiatrists take their cue from normative social behaviour, despite best efforts to remain dispassionate and impartial, they cannot escape making value judgements. For example, the diagnosis of personality disorder puts a medical label on human behaviour that is at variance with the 'norm'. Yet what

---

2. Rogers (1989: 27).
3. For a well-argued rebuttal of the materialist view that the mind is nothing but a product of the brain, see *Open Sciences Manifesto* (Open Sciences, 2014).
4. William Shakespeare: *Hamlet*. Hamlet to Horatio (Act 1, scene 5, lines 167–168).

evidence do we have for saying personality disorder is either an illness or a disease?

Being a competent and caring psychiatrist is probably one of the hardest jobs around. Most psychiatrists – myself included – take up the specialty because they are deeply interested in human nature and genuinely wish to help their patients find relief from inordinate suffering. Yet it behoves us to leaf through a few pages of history to see what our profession has been doing.

My generation of psychiatrists, trained in the 1970s, was emboldened by the twin pillars of research at the time, depth psychology and pharmacotherapy, to think that most mental illnesses would respond to one or other approach. Since then, there has been a proliferation of psychological and pharmaceutical treatments. Neuroscience has begun to map brain function in ways that were unimaginable 20 years ago and research continues apace into genetic and epigenetic vulnerability to mental disorder, covert neurodevelopmental abnormalities, the physiological sequelae of emotional trauma on the brain, biochemical triggers and the impact of substance misuse. The list is long and ever lengthening.

I dare say academic psychiatrists pore over the many research papers (with their formidable statistics) found these days in publications such as the *British Journal of Psychiatry*. Yet most psychiatrists I know would admit to simply scanning the headlines to see if something there might help with a problem in the clinic. The sacred cow of large-scale outcome research seems a long way off when one is faced with the patient as a unique individual, on whom stresses are impacting in a unique way.

The problem is that while year on year the research database proliferates, less and less of it seems to be about person-centred care. A moment's reflection on the history of pharmaceutical 'breakthroughs' is instructive, for boundless initial optimism has so often turned out to be seriously misplaced. The 1960s saw the disastrous prescribing of benzodiazepines and the subsequent misery of long-term addiction for vast numbers of people.[5] At around the same time, monoamine oxidase inhibitors (MAOIs) succeeded tricyclic antidepressants as the new wonder drugs until the risk of potentially fatal hypertensive crisis curtailed their use. Another surge of enthusiasm heralded the arrival of the selective serotonin reuptake inhibitors (SSRIs) in the 1990s. Now, the many serious side-effects of SSRIs are increasingly being recognised.[6]

---

5. Even today, despite clear warnings that the maximum duration should be no more than one month, there are over 250,000 patients in the UK taking benzodiazepines prescribed by their general practitioner for longer than a year. See Davies et al. (2017).
6. For a full and sobering review, see Andrews et al. (2012).

It is not known whether these medications help speed recovery or whether they merely provide a degree of symptom relief until the passage of time enables recovery to take place. Meanwhile, the pharmacotherapy of psychosis remains deeply problematic. First-generation phenothiazines caused serious neurological side-effects, sometimes permanently, and subsequent generations of antipsychotics have also produced a range of adverse reactions. More recently, evidence suggests that while short-term use of antipsychotics can help, long-term medication actually worsens prognosis.[7]

The burden of disability in mental healthcare is enormous. Schizophrenia and bipolar disorder each have a worldwide prevalence of 1–2%. With a world population aged 15 upwards of over 5 billion, the sum total of those affected comes to more than 100 million. Many psychiatrists believe that these two conditions are caused by physical and/or neurochemical abnormalities in the brain, although the evidence is at best patchy.[8] Then there is all the rest, a great melting pot of psychopathology, symptomatology, morbidity and complex presentations of personal, interpersonal and social dysfunction.

In the high-income world, we have a veritable epidemic of depression on our hands. According to the World Health Organization, the prevalence of depression worldwide totals over 300 million at any one time, with 800,000 suicides a year (after accidents, now the second most common cause of death in 15- to 29-year-olds).[9] Neither are the young spared – around one child in ten in the USA is being medicated for attention deficit hyperactivity disorder.[10]

Substance misuse is also of epidemic proportions. In the UK, one adult in thirteen is dependent on alcohol, with 8500 deaths per year directly attributable to alcohol[11] and over 21,000 deaths through illness associated with habitual alcohol misuse (more than 1 million such hospital admissions per year).[12] As for illicit drugs, these days 10% of the UK population are using them, leading to a further 2500 deaths per year.[13]

---

7. Insel (2013).
8. Recent brain studies of patients with schizophrenia have suggested a loss of cell volume in the hippocampus, a neural structure in the temporal lobe of the brain, although the significance is not yet clear. Allen (2016).
9. World Health Organization (2017).
10. Visser et al. (2014).
11. Office for National Statistics (2014).
12. Alcohol Concern (2016).
13. Office for National Statistics (2015).

The magnitude of the mental health problem is such that some 20% of patients seeing their general practitioner are suffering from an emotional disorder and up to another 20% from somatoform disorders including chronic fatigue, musculoskeletal and chronic pain disorders, palpitations, functional gastrointestinal symptoms, body dysmorphophobia and hypochondriasis.[14]

What does an epidemic of mental illness such as this signify? Can this really be some new kind of biological disorder afflicting the human race? I hardly think so! How much of it is the sheer culmination of misery that goes with the human condition, but not previously labelled with a diagnosis? How much more arises from the cultural changes of the past 100 years, in which material success and consumerism have become new gods at the cost of impoverishment of the inner life?

The Role of the Psychiatrist

We know that stress can bring about changes in brain chemistry, some probably irreversible and leading to long-term vulnerability to illness.[15] I am certain we will never understand mental illness by looking at it in isolation; rather, we must look at the whole person and their life context. For example, in our consumerist world, geared to the young nuclear family, ageing is for many a lonely and disheartening prospect. Little awaits most elderly people except the prospect of disability, often with dementia and ending their lives in a care home or hospital bed. It is hardly surprising that the prevalence of depression in the over 65s is more than 25%.[16] People need to be in relationship with other people from cradle to grave. Mental illness, whatever the age and diagnosis, only increases this basic need. Yet in the 'developed countries' the picture is frequently one of isolation. Clearly, no pharmaceutical treatment will remedy this.

How about psychotherapy? Unfortunately, because of financial pressures on the service, mainstream therapies are now short-term. Where is the time and opportunity to establish a trusting and dependable human relationship in order to help the patient explore a new and better future, and to accompany them a while on their new path?

---

14. For full discussion, see Royal College of Psychiatrists & Royal College of General Practitioners (2009).
15. Chetty et al. (2014).
16. An estimated 85% of the over 65s receive no support or treatment. See Mental Health Foundation (2006).

A further pressure on psychiatry is in balancing the role of physician with that of social policeman. There are serious ethical issues here. To what extent has the psychiatrist the right to assume responsibility for another person? Is someone intent on taking their life invariably deemed to be ill and therefore to be rescued from themselves? Further, what is the meaning of risk? Should psychiatrists necessarily fall in with the social norms of a risk-averse society?

In the UK 40 years ago, things seemed more straightforward. Even though the treatment might not work, at least it seemed we knew what we were doing – after all, treatments do not always work in general medicine either. The psychiatric establishment brushed aside the radical theories of the psychiatrist R.D. Laing[17,18] and busied itself with demonstrating that the mental health profession could stand shoulder to shoulder with any other branch of medicine. This optimism was harnessed by the UK government initiative of closing down mental hospitals in favour of 'care in the community'.[19] Unfortunately, lack of resources seriously hampered good intentions and many patients ended up isolated and living alone.

The old-style medical model was now being superseded by the multidisciplinary team approach. Surely, this would lead to more compassionate, rounded and person-centred provision of mental healthcare? Yet for some patients, this approach did not work so well. Formerly, the consultant psychiatrist had been indisputably in charge. Patients were offered an illness model that relieved uncertainty and was delivered with conviction. A patient was 'under' Dr So-and-so, who maintained personal contact, often for many years. Consultants knew their patients much like the old-fashioned general practitioner and this greatly reassured some service users – at least those who were fortunate to be looked after by a conscientious psychiatrist.

Although well intended, the new-style multidisciplinary team also introduced a good deal of unintended confusion. The familiarity and informality with which a whole range of staff would meet and greet patients offered friendly support but did not guarantee any deeper understanding. Patients compulsorily treated under the Mental Health Act could find themselves in a Kafkaesque scenario. Who is staff (no dress code)? How are decisions being made? How to tell nurse from doctor?

---

17. Laing (1970).
18. Laing & Esterson (1970).
19. The National Health Service and Community Care Act of 1990 created an internal market for the supply of healthcare, transferring responsibility for provision of health and social care to local authorities.

As pressure on beds increased, in-patient units increasingly became places of containment for seriously and acutely ill patients. Gone was the notion of admission to hospital as a relief from stress, a sanctuary that for some people had been a valued provision of care. The 'patient journey' as it was now called, came to be accompanied by a bewildering array of support agencies and healthcare staff. Yet who among them had both the motivation and time to reach out and connect with the personhood of the patient?

From Pathology to Personhood

My own specialisation in psychotherapy at the Maudsley Hospital, London, took me into the world of psychoanalysis. This ensured that I continued working at a deep level with my patients, which was a source of great personal satisfaction for me. Nevertheless, as the years passed, I began to question the nature of the clinical set-up, with its strange formality, the focus on unconscious defence and the imbalance of power consequent on the inevitable dynamics that arise. I also saw that if the therapist keeps their patient too long in treatment, the patient could as easily get buried in their childhood as freed from it.

Subsequent training as a group analyst took me into the more egalitarian setting of the therapeutic group. The members of the group come from very different backgrounds and share in their varied life experience, importantly giving each other support while challenging the others' assumptions and behaviours. As the group develops and matures, members learn to value and affirm each other's personhood – not blindly, but with growing discernment.

Nevertheless, the dynamics that surface in the group cannot help but constellate the group as a family, with the therapist effectively in the parent role or with co-therapists as a parental couple. After a number of years, I began to feel I had been a professional parent for long enough.

I later trained in psychodrama, where I found the climate of democracy appealing and refreshing. The therapist (director) helps guide the patient (protagonist) through scenes from life, chosen by the patient and enacted for therapeutic purposes. Most scenes are about crucial events in the past, but potential future scenes may be rehearsed too. Group members take on the roles of important 'others', chosen by the patient/protagonist when recreating the situation to be explored.

The therapist/director studiously avoids interpreting what is in the mind of the protagonist, or presuming to know what should be worked on next; it is for the protagonist to choose what and whom to face.

Often feelings that previously had to be suppressed erupt with full force. In scenes of heartfelt loss, the protagonist may need to be physically held and comforted, an experience that sometimes breaks through a lifetime of isolation. At the conclusion of the session, the group members, including the therapist, spend time sharing how they felt affected by taking part and how it touched on their own lives. The mutual support and concern for each other builds trust and restores hope.

The importance of addressing personhood was brought home to me by my work in psychodrama, yet validating personhood does not require a particular therapeutic approach. It is only necessary for the clinician to remember at all times that we are much more like our patients than we are different, and that they deserve to be shown the same respect, care and compassion that we would wish for ourselves.

Personhood and Recovery

It has been stated by William Anthony that in cases of severe mental illness ongoing symptoms do not need to hinder 'recovery' provided that the person experiences a way of living that is satisfying, hopeful and contributing to life, even with limitations caused by illness.[20] To this, we might add a pithy observation by Professor Larry Davidson from Yale, who says,

> 'Recovery means learning how to live outside the mental illness rather than inside it. To live inside the mental illness is to be lost in its downward spiral. Living outside schizophrenia is about reclaiming your life. It is about self-determination, choice, hope, and empowerment'.[21]

This is an important statement, one that we should not limit to schizophrenia, for it addresses the danger of a person becoming identified with their 'illness' – living inside it and even being defined by it. A label can purport to explain everything when, in truth, it explains little or nothing. Every time the mental health professional reiterates the diagnosis, identification with the sick role is reinforced. Little wonder we hear young adults report having had 'depression' sometimes for 10 years or more. Depression, in particular, has come to be worn like a badge – often getting in the way of taking a fresh look at what is really going on.

The injunction to 'live outside your illness' has universal application, for illness of one kind or another will cast its shadow on everyone at

---

20. Anthony (1993).
21. Summerville (2009).

some time. Confusion, pain and loss go with the actuality of life. The challenge that faces us all is to take responsibility for living the best life we can that circumstances will allow. Learning how to assume responsibility for oneself and one's life, whatever it may bring, is at the heart of personhood.

This issue is crucial in mental healthcare. Sometimes psychiatrists are obliged to intervene and force a person along a path not chosen – for example, compulsory admission to hospital under the Mental Health Act. Although the intervention may be necessary, it understandably inculcates resentment and resistance. There is the world of difference between encouragement and coercion; where the former affirms personhood, the latter diminishes it, something that good psychiatric practice requires we never forget.

From Personhood to Soul

Psychodrama brought home to me the awareness of how much we are all fellow travellers in life, sharing in the same challenges, struggles and growing pains that beset every human being. Moreover, I saw something else that impressed me deeply – that when a person takes on the role of someone they perceive as good and wise, they find themselves speaking from within that role with wisdom beyond their experience and years.

How had I missed seeing that before? The most likely answer is that psychiatry does not expect patients to have the wherewithal, for the patient is taken to be unwell and the psychiatrist is there to diagnose and treat. Mainstream psychotherapy makes a similar assumption, since the therapist has studied the workings of the mind, including unconscious processes of which the patient is unaware, and is generally perceived by both of them as being the wiser and more knowing.

From psychodrama, I went on to make myself familiar with the writings of Carl Jung and his researches into the archetypes, in particular the Self, which Jung describes as the supreme archetype of the collective unconscious.[22] The Self imparts a subtle knowledge of things

---

22. The term *archetype* refers to an inherited idea or mode of thought that has its source in the collective unconscious of humankind. Archetypes are expressed as images or personifications. The Self to which Jung refers stands for the totality of the psyche (personal and transpersonal) in which the Imago Dei (the God-image) is pre-eminent. Jung writes '[It] pervades the whole human sphere and makes mankind its involuntary exponent...' (1958: 417).

greater than the everyday world of the egoic self, a grand, transcendent perspective that is the birthright of every human being.

Accordingly, when we listen to the soul, we are taken beyond the mundane level of social habits, needs and desires. We find ourselves seeking meaning and purpose in a larger framework, one that encompasses birth, life and death. This is not the 'ungrounded' kind of spirituality that leads to turning away from human friendship and society. Rather, a person feels able to experience and express themselves authentically, both inwardly – the imaginal world – and outwardly in relation to others. To be able to live wholeheartedly becomes more important than striving for the conventional trappings of worldly success.

Psychodrama had taken me outside mainstream psychotherapy and I never really went back. Instead, I became deeply interested in transpersonal psychology and began learning more about soul-centred therapies. At first, I hesitated to use the word 'soul' in clinical practice. Yet what else should I call the innate wisdom that can be brought to bear on the trials and tribulations of the ego while remaining untouched by the storms of life – and with a depth of insight that goes even beyond personhood?

Left to its own devices, the human mind deals with intractable problems by labelling them and then usually agonising about them. Unfortunately, the mind can tell itself just about anything and since it has very little sense of direction, a person is liable to find themselves being buffeted by storm force winds. Because the ego identifies so strongly with its own subjective pursuits, the larger context is missing – one that would keep things in proportion. Consequently, the ego behaves like the star performer on the stage of life, writing the script, building the sets and props, insisting on taking centre-stage and then, when things go wrong, blaming the play for being somebody else's creation!

On the other hand, when we let ourselves be guided by the soul, we are better able to discern the problem for what it truly is. This is not to treat the problem as unimportant, but to maintain equanimity and clear-sightedness when they are most needed.

From the perspective of the soul, what the ego takes to be love is very often need in disguise, and when needs are frustrated, anger is kindled. Then we really start to suffer, and make others suffer too. In contrast, soul awareness is characterised by an emanation of love that feels deeply for the oneness of humanity. Love of this nature asks for nothing in return, knowing only the desire to help and to heal. When personhood is under threat, the soul's unfailing desire is to help restore wholeness of being and magnanimity of heart.

Mindful of the Soul

In this paper, I have wanted to bring out the importance of seeking the counsel of the soul, especially when suffering the pain of breakdown. Further, since we need to know what to be looking for in order to find it, I have characterised the soul with a description that falls woefully short, but which I hope is sufficient to remind us of its constant presence.

I have written at some length elsewhere how soul awareness can be engaged by means of specific therapeutic approaches.[23] Here I want to conclude by highlighting something else, which owes nothing to a particular method or technique, requires no psychotherapy training and applies to the whole field of mental healthcare – as indeed it should to every human relationship. Nevertheless, it is frequently overlooked because it does not suit the ego to remember it.

Only by the example we set do we inspire others to do likewise. Patients who are simply diagnosed and treated like case studies from a textbook will never reveal themselves. If, however, while addressing our patients' mental health needs we set out to engage with their personhood, we will both get to know the patient and affirm the person. If we go the extra mile and trust the soul to guide us in our work, we find our patients will respond to us soul to soul. This does not have to mean a lot of talking, but being 'present' in such a way that our patients feel the depth of our genuine respect and understanding, and our willingness to face the unknown with them.

When we offer this, we facilitate a depth of connection and a breadth of vision that transcends the wounds of the ego. To borrow from the words of Reinhold Niebuhr,[24] we are thereby helped to find the serenity to accept the things we cannot change, courage to change the things we can, and wisdom to know the difference.

As the soul does not pass judgement, our patients will not feel judged. Because the soul is compassionate, our patients will be helped to forgive themselves and others. And, because the soul knows only love, our patients are helped to heal.

---

23. See *Soul-Centred Psychotherapy* and *Open Heart, Open Mind: Conversing with the Soul*, this volume.
24. Niebuhr's 'serenity prayer': 'God grant me the serenity to accept the things I cannot change; courage to change the things I can; and wisdom to know the difference'. In Zaleski & Zaleski (2005: 127).

References

Andrews, P., Thomson, J., Amstadter, A., et al. (2012) *Primum non nocere*: an evolutionary analysis of whether antidepressants do more harm than good. *Frontiers in Psychology*, 24 April.

Alcohol Concern (2016) Alcohol statistics. Available at: https://www.alcoholconcern.org.uk/alcohol-statistics (accessed 8 July 2017).

Allen, K., Fung, S. & Weickert, C. (2016) Cell proliferation is reduced in the hippocampus in schizophrenia. *Australian and New Zealand Journal of Psychiatry*, 50, 473–480.

Anthony, W.A. (1993) Recovery from mental illness: the guiding vision of the mental health service system in the 1990s. *Psychosocial Rehabilitation Journal*, 16, 11–23.

Chetty, S., Friedman, A., Taravosh-Lahn, K., et al. (2014) Stress and glucocorticoids promote oligodendrogenesis in the adult hippocampus. *Molecular Psychiatry*, 19, 1275–1283.

Davies, J., Rae, T.C. & Montagu, L. (2017) Long-term benzodiazepine and Z-drugs use in the UK: a survey of general practice. *British Journal of General Practice*, 67, 609–613.

Insel, T. (2013) Antipsychotics: taking the long view [blog]. Available at: https://www.nimh.nih.gov/about/directors/thomas-insel/blog/2013/antipsychotics-taking-the-long-view.shtml (accessed 4 July 2017).

Jung, C.G. (1958) Answer to Job. In *C.G. Jung: The Collected Works*, vol. 11, Psychology and Religion: West and East (eds H. Read, M. Fordham & G. Adler). Routledge and Kegan Paul.

Laing, R. (1970) *The Divided Self*. Pelican.

Laing, R. & Esterson, A. (1970) *Sanity, Madness and the Family*. Penguin Books.

Mental Health Foundation (2006) Mental health statistics: older people. Mental Health Foundation. Available at: https://www.mentalhealth.org.uk/statistics/mental-health-statistics-older-people (accessed 10 September 2017).

Office for National Statistics (2014) Alcohol related deaths in the United Kingdom: 2014 registrations. ONS. Available at: https://www.ons.gov.uk/peoplepopulationandcommunity/healthandsocialcare/causesofdeath/bulletins/alcoholrelateddeathsintheunitedkingdom/registeredin2014 (accessed 8 July 2017).

Office for National Statistics (2015) Deaths related to drug poisoning in England and Wales: 2015 registrations. ONS. Available at: https://www.ons.gov.uk/peoplepopulationandcommunity/birthsdeathsandmarriages/deaths/bulletins/deathsrelatedtodrugpoisoninginenglandandwales/2015registrations#main-points (accessed 8 July 2017).

Open Sciences (2014) Manifesto for a Post-Materialist Science. Campaign for Open Science. Available at: http://opensciences.org/about/manifesto-for-a-post-materialist-science (accessed 8 July 2017).

Rogers, C. (1989) *The Carl Rogers Reader* (eds H. Kirschenbaum & V.L. Henderson). Howard Mifflin.

Royal College of Psychiatrists & Royal College of General Practitioners (2009) *The Management of Patients with Physical and Psychological Problems in Primary Care: A Practical Guide* (College Report CR152). RCPsych. Available at: http://www.rcpsych.ac.uk/files/pdfversion/CR152x.pdf (accessed 8 July 2017).

Summerville, C. (2009) Your Recovery Journey: Message from CEO. Your Recovery Journey. Available at: http://www.your-recovery-journey.ca/Message.htm (accessed 8 July 2017).

Visser, S., Danielson, M., Bitsko, R., et al. (2014) Trends in the parent-report of health care provider-diagnosed and medicated ADHD: United States, 2003–2011. *Journal of the American Academy of Child and Adolescent Psychiatry*, 53, 34–46.

World Health Organization (2014) Mental health: a state of well-being. Fact file update. WHO. Available at: http://www.who.int/features/factfiles/mental_health/en/ (accessed 8 July 2017).

World Health Organization (2017) Factsheet on depression. WHO. Available at: http://www.who.int/mediacentre/factsheets/fs369/en/ (accessed 8 July 2017).

Zaleski, P. & Zaleski, C. (2005) *Prayer: A History*. Houghton Mifflin.

10

Vocation Under Duress

'Be the change your wish to see happen
instead of trying to change anyone else.'[1]

To be a good clinician entails coping with diagnostic uncertainty, complex risk management and inadequate resources. It also calls for the capacity to remain open-hearted and empathic. Regrettably, these days many people in the UK view the National Health Service (NHS) with apprehension and even distrust. In this paper I will be exploring how we may respond to the needs of the institution and its staff when morale is in decline and goodwill is in short supply.

First, I will review some of the changes I have seen during my professional lifetime. Second, I will discuss the current crisis in the NHS with particular reference to Abraham Maslow's 'hierarchy of needs'. Lastly, I will suggest how, by drawing on Maslow's conceptual framework, we might remedy some of the deficits and their impact on healthcare staff.

Early Days

The NHS was created in 1948 by Aneurin Bevan, then Minister of Health, based on the ideal that good healthcare should be freely available to all. In the immediate post-war years the NHS acted as a unifying social force, one in which everyone could take pride.

Paper prepared for conference 'Furthering Kindness and Kinship in Mental Healthcare', held by the Spirituality and Psychiatry Special Interest Group at the Royal College of Psychiatrists, London, April 2013.

---

1. Often attributed to Mahatma Gandhi, although the authorship is more likely Arleen Lorrance (2001: 105–118).

When I became a doctor in 1969, medical technology was generally affordable. Patients did not question their treatments, taking on trust what was offered, and when things went wrong did not generally blame it on doctors or nurses. Mistakes were doubtless made and were probably more easily concealed. Nevertheless, I am describing a time when doctors had the confidence of their patients.

Senior nursing sisters with long years of experience ran hospital wards. The relationship between the ward sister and the consultant was crucial. They were, archetypally, mother and father presiding over a drama of life and death, sometimes curing, more often alleviating and other times helping people die as good a death as could be managed.

As a young hospital doctor, I remember admitting a man in his forties with a brainstem stroke. He was motionless and seemingly unconscious but while examining him, I noticed that his eyes, which were open and staring ahead, had a look of alertness about them. I asked him to blink if he could hear me. He not only heard me but could understand as well. He was otherwise entirely paralysed, known today as locked-in syndrome.[2]

On the ward round, I told my consultant what I had found. He took the man's hand, gave a nod to the ward sister and said to the patient kindly, 'I'll come and have a chat with you later'. I started early the next morning and finding the bed empty, I asked Sister about it. She deliberated, looked me in the eye and quietly said, 'He passed away in the night'. Instinctively, I felt I knew what may have happened.

There is a fierce debate, these days more than ever, about the rights and wrongs of assisted suicide. Those against it will see in this story exactly why it should never be allowed. If my supposition was correct, others will read into it the humanity of a doctor caring for his critically ill patient in accordance with a person's wishes. There were bad people around before Harold Shipman, the general practitioner found guilty of serial murders in 2000, but they did not influence the practice of medicine in those times.

Behind the consultant and ward sister stood the hospital itself, the 'Stone Mother', as Henri Rey, a psychoanalyst who later supervised me at the Maudsley Hospital, called it. Patients with intractable conditions, whether physical or emotional, could rely on this 'mother'. While

---

2. In cases of the locked-in syndrome it is extremely rare for any motor recovery to take place. However, in recent years, with increased awareness of the syndrome, the medico-legal duty of care is to provide life support with the use of digital devices to aid communication. This can sometimes mean being committed to the ongoing treatment of a patient who constantly asks to be released from their misery. Other patients are more accepting of their condition, as in the powerful personal narrative recorded by Bauby (1998).

doctors might come and go, 'she' could be counted on to stay and be entirely dependable.

These days the Stone Mother is not so dependable, as the Health Commission inquiry into mortality rates at Stafford Hospital has revealed.[3] Across the UK, hospital-acquired infections are running at 10%, many of them resistant to antibiotics. Side-effects of medication, dispensing mistakes and surgical errors of judgement accounted for nearly 3000 hospital deaths in the UK in 2013.[4]

Changing Times

After taking the membership examination of the Royal College of Physicians, I began my training in psychiatry at the Maudsley and Bethlem hospitals. I observed that many patients were admitted because they needed sanctuary from whatever it was that was making them ill. As in general hospitals at the time, the decision to admit was made by the consultant, without administrators, as they were then called, questioning the need. These days a patient has to be very ill, most likely psychotic, to be admitted to an in-patient unit, where the high level of disturbance is hardly conducive to respite.

Those were also the dying days of the large mental hospitals, some of which I remember visiting. 'Care in the community'[5] had become the new mantra and had much to commend it, if only it could be properly resourced and managed. Unfortunately, as it turned out, there was a cost; a drab and lonely future awaited many of the long-stay patients for whom the institution had become home. Those asylums had been strange and surreal places, yet a kindness was to be found among many of the staff, who understood that sometimes patients were helped most by accepting them the way they were and in providing them with a familiar and safe environment in which to live.

While at the Maudsley, I was briefly seconded to Dr Douglas Bennett at St. Francis' Hospital in Dulwich, where something of the old-style ambience remained. The main ward area was locked, yet no one seemed particularly at risk and the nurse in charge, always wearing a large bunch of keys, readily let patients in and out. I decided to hold a large group meeting to discuss this issue. The patients and nurses all came, and Douglas Bennett too. To my surprise, the patients voted to

---

3. Francis (2013).
4. Campbell (2013).
5. Consequent on the National Health Service and Community Care Act 1990.

keep the door locked. We generally put a lock on our own front doors and I rather think these patients felt the same way.

At the Maudsley Hospital, there were no white coats and the nurses dressed casually, a trend that was becoming the norm for mental health services. Years later, as a visiting consultant to other units, I found it was sometimes difficult to tell who was staff, since a dress code of shirt and jeans was commonplace. On ringing the ward, the phone might be answered with a breezy 'hallo', and just the first name proffered, without it being clear who was actually in charge.

It struck me at the same time that doctors no longer held the same authority. Multidisciplinary teams were being established, with lead nurses and consultant clinical psychologists now taking referrals. Some psychiatrists privately voiced concerns about being held responsible for patients they never saw.

I was interested in this ceding of authority, not because I hold that authority is sacrosanct, but because I wondered what kind of health service we were heading for. The shift had started during the late 1980s, while I was still a consultant at St George's Hospital in London. Under the benign guidance of Professor Arthur Crisp, we enjoyed a golden decade for psychiatry. We had been able to strengthen clinical services with new consultant appointments and to set up a number of accredited higher specialist trainings. Then a new tier of administration began to impose serious constraints on funding. Lengthy documents began to appear on our desks, punctuated with business-speak about the need for income generation and efficiency measures. This was before email, so we waded through the pages and tried to absorb what it meant for our service.

Demoralisation Sets In

This was a point at which we consultants could probably have continued to run the show, had we the stomach for dealing with cuts to services. However, we had never envisaged having to wrangle with each other over resources and we did not like it. The government of the day, driven by political imperatives and exasperated with what it saw as resistance to change, began to set up trusts. Consultants soon realised that they no longer held the same authority.

I recall one trivial incident, symbolic of the changing times. I had by now moved to Oxford and happened to be visiting a patient at the nearby John Radcliffe Hospital. To my surprise and irritation, I suddenly found that my NHS car parking permit no longer worked at the John Radcliffe, for overnight it had become an independent trust. Not long after, we psychiatrists found ourselves part of a similarly new mental health trust.

Before these changes, being a doctor in the NHS had felt like belonging to one big family that pulled together through thick and thin. Now we were following the American model of turning medicine into a business for which trusts would soon be competing. Managers, whose horizons were financial, came on the scene with little or no experience of medical services and for whom patients were numbers on a page. Some doctors became medical directors, hoping to bridge the divide and do some good, but often found themselves viewed with suspicion by clinical colleagues. An era of grievance had begun.

The Hierarchy of Needs

Over the past 20 years, psychiatry has benefited from advances in neuroscience, together with new pharmacological and psychological approaches. So why should morale remain poor, why do staff feel burdened and why does it fall to charities like the Mental Health Foundation to headline the need for forward-planning in order to meet the growing level of mental ill health?[6]

In looking at what may have led to this problem of disaffection and low morale, I am going to draw on the work of the psychologist Abraham Maslow and his 'hierarchy of needs'. The term was introduced in Maslow's paper 'A theory of Human Motivation'[7] and can be represented schematically:

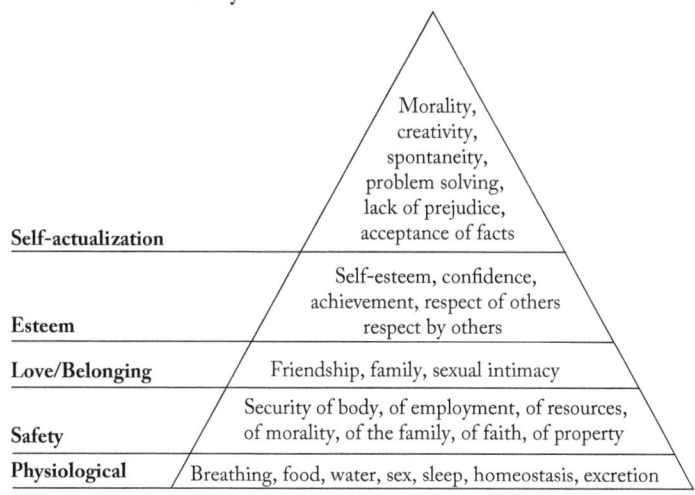

Self-actualization	Morality, creativity, spontaneity, problem solving, lack of prejudice, acceptance of facts
Esteem	Self-esteem, confidence, achievement, respect of others, respect by others
Love/Belonging	Friendship, family, sexual intimacy
Safety	Security of body, of employment, of resources, of morality, of the family, of faith, of property
Physiological	Breathing, food, water, sex, sleep, homeostasis, excretion

10.1. Maslow's hierarchy of needs.[8]

---

6. Mental Health Foundation (2016).
7. Maslow (1943).
8. From image by J. Finklestein (2006) and released under license by Wikimedia Commons.

The hierarchy is usually shown as a pyramid, although Maslow himself never described it as such. According to Maslow, each level has to rest securely on the firm foundation of the level below.

Physiological survival comes first, then the need for safety, both physical and emotional, before we are in a position to love and value others and ourselves. Then it becomes possible to engage with real intimacy in relationships and, beyond that, to contribute to what is best in humankind.[9]

The First Level: Care of the Body

As house officers (the most junior medical appointments), my generation of young doctors regularly worked 120 hours a week, entailing residential on-call every other night as well as normal daytime duties. We lived on enthusiasm and deep loyalty to the NHS. Since that time, studies have shown that judgement becomes seriously impaired due to sleep deprivation, with alarming loss of insight. However, even today, many hospital doctors still work week-long shifts of 90 hours, despite the limit of 48 hours set down by the European Working Time Directive.

The military know from training exercises that a group of people left to forage for themselves for just three days will start off companionably enough, but soon any conversation that remains is reduced to finding something to eat and keeping warm – such is the nature of survival mentality. I am reminded of the working lunches to which we consultants became inured – a cold sandwich with a cup of lukewarm coffee from an urn – while we ploughed our way through new business plans, always with the shadow of cuts, now called efficiency savings, hanging over us. We were no longer planning new services but trying to hang on to what we already had. The enlivening chance to share work concerns in friendly and informal exchanges was slipping away.

These privations, however, were nothing compared with failures of patient care that have since come to light. The frail elderly are especially at risk, the Care Quality Commission (CQC) having found that 20% of hospitals in the UK do not provide adequate facilities.[10]

In 2013, the shocking contents of the Francis Report were published in detail. To quote:

> '…patients were left lying in soiled sheeting and sitting on commodes for hours… left unwashed, at times for up to a month… forced to rely

---

9. Throughout history, the great spiritual masters are portrayed as having eschewed the more usual human needs represented by Maslow's schema.
10. Care Quality Commission (2011).

on family members for help with feeding... pain relief was provided late or in some cases not at all... families were forced to remove used bandages and dressings from public areas and clean the toilets themselves'.

Mental healthcare patients are highly vulnerable too, as was found in the case of the Winterbourne View Care Home, exposed by the BBC television programme *Panorama* in 2011.[11] Brutal systematic abuse of young adults with learning disabilities and challenging behaviour was revealed, resulting in a full-scale government inquiry.[12]

Individuals responsible for abuse need holding to account. Yet, as in the days of the Third Reich, people who might otherwise be regarded as decent enough can get drawn in by sanctioned sadism. In a culture of brutal indifference, low-paid, poorly trained care workers – traditionally the underdogs – seize the chance to wield power. Truth may be the first casualty of war but altruism is the first casualty of privation.

The Second Level: Safety and Security

The importance of safety and security for self and one's kith and kin cannot be overstated. Feeling under threat triggers the physiology of the fight/flight response, intended by Nature to last no more than about twenty minutes before returning to the resting state. Chronic high levels of stress, where the only option is to soldier on, have been shown to be highly injurious to both mind and body. Enforced stoicism, especially when carrying responsibility for others without the means to take effective action, leads to cardiovascular disease, anxiety, depression and burnout.

In 2001, one in five doctors was planning early retirement. By 2008, this had risen to over one-third and today the numbers are higher still. Those who stay and fight for better conditions take a big risk, for whistle-blowers have been summarily suspended or pensioned off with gagging clauses. Between 2010 and 2013, 15 million pounds was spent by trusts dealing in this way with over 600 complainants.[13]

Now that much of this is coming into the open, the danger is that trusts will be vilified without an understanding of how the same persecutory dynamics apply to managers. Government directives squeeze the managers to put targets before people, targets that often cannot realistically be met. Consequently, managers live in fear of failure, fear of loss of funding, fear of being blamed for everything that goes wrong, and fear of losing their livelihoods.

---

11. BBC One (2011).
12. Department of Health (2012).
13. Pierce (2013).

At the same time, the cost of healthcare is spiralling, not only due to state-of-the-art technologies but also on account of the increasing burden of pathology and care needs that accompany greater longevity. Since resources can never catch up with demand, managers continue to pile on the pressure as they try to square the circle.

This leads to scapegoating. The dynamic is as follows: the irksome problem is disowned and gets projected elsewhere, best done by finding someone or something to blame. Thereby, denial of responsibility allows for preservation of self-esteem, however shaky it may be. At the same time, handing on blame is like passing around a bomb with a slow fuse. Doctors blame managers; managers blame government (and doctors); government blames the legacy of debt left by the opposition; the opposition does its utmost to persecute the government, which then comes up with some new system (such as general practitioner-led commissioning groups). Next, it turns out that one-third of general practitioners are found to have conflicting financial interests when undertaking commissioning. The General Medical Council requires new powers to monitor this and in doing so, becomes another persecutor to add to the mix.

The Third Level: Love and Belonging

Next in Maslow's hierarchy come the primary social needs of friendship, family and sexual intimacy. However, it should be noted that for love to be managed appropriately and responsibly, the need for safety must first have been established. Otherwise, as in the case of the paedophile Jimmy Savile,[14] perverse and predatory behaviour can thrive in institutional settings that offer both opportunity and concealment.

Here I want to enlarge for a moment on the archetype of the family and the bonds of kinship, for they evoke strong emotions that originated early in life – when there was a group of just two, mother and infant. Even then, the wider group was present (although once removed), for also acting on the mother were the key relationships she internalised from her own childhood and which she unconsciously presents to her baby. Then there is the influence of the baby's father, other family and friends, and often day care too, all shaping a child's encounter with the first big institution – school. Some children shrink

---

14. Savile was a popular radio and television personality in the UK and a charity fundraiser who gained high-profile access to schools, hospitals and other institutions. After Savile's death, he was discovered to have sexually abused hundreds of children. See Lampard & Marsden (2015).

back, some throw themselves into the fray, while others stand on the side-lines, more inclined to become observers of human nature.

In adult life, institutions continue to attract a strong emotional charge, for how each person responds to the culture of the institution will be coloured by the kind of relationships they experienced during their early development – whether accepting or rejecting, tolerant or demanding, caring or indifferent. That is the one half; the other half, of course, concerns how in actuality the institution behaves.

The generation of doctors to which I belonged may have been politically naive, but we shared an ideal for an NHS that we held in real affection, one that cared for us while we did our best to care for our patients. The kinship was like an extended family and was nationwide, extending to doctors, nurses, the emergency services and ancillary staff, not least hospital porters.

While I was an undergraduate at Cambridge, I worked as a porter at Addenbrooke's Hospital during one summer vacation. It was an upstairs–downstairs world, in which we porters were ensconced in the bowels of the hospital. Apart from moving patients around and delivering mail, porters had to incinerate the hospital waste. We knew that without us, the hospital could not last a day. Yet how many doctors were ever likely to think about that? Nevertheless, up in the corridors of power, if a doctor or nurse gave a nod of recognition to an approaching porter, we felt seen and valued. Feeling part of the family depended on such small and very human moments. Happily, most of the staff was friendly, and so were we.

Even without the rose-tint of nostalgia, this third level of Maslow's has a lot to say about the medical world of the 1970s and 1980s. Technology had not interposed between people as it does today. In a world without email, we talked to each other more, and consequently, we understood each other and liked each other better. Years later, when decision-making became the province of trust management, the edicts issued from on high, no matter how laudable, never felt owned by the people expected to carry them out.

The Fourth Level: Esteem and Respect

Maslow's fourth level is characterised by a shift from the personal to the interpersonal. This is the healthy outcome for mature selfhood when anxious preoccupations have been surmounted. Holding self and others in esteem is a precondition to the healthy functioning of any institution. Problems that arise are not driven by personal agendas and so there is no need for scapegoating. People are better able to see things as they really are, feel more confident of their own sovereignty and – perhaps because they do not feel under threat – are genuinely more open to others. When people enjoy being together, feeling connected and helped to do what they are good at, more work gets done.

I used to run staff groups in various mental healthcare settings. Group morale was always a key concern. Sometimes we could usefully explore staff problems that were getting in the way of patient care. On the other hand, if a problem had its source elsewhere in the institution, trying to contain it in the group would risk colluding with the institution.

Steve Denning, a pioneer in the field of 'radical management', emphasises the primacy of the need for connectedness and re-draws Maslow's schema thus:

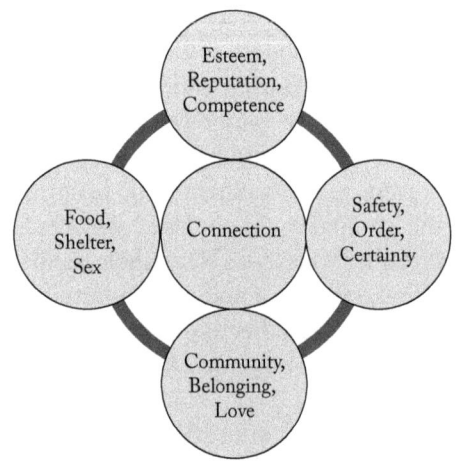

10.2 Interlocking systems of radical management.[15]

Denning argues for a move away from top-down bureaucracy towards self-organising teams that foster values and innovative solutions. This is the ethos of Silicon Valley, California, very different from reliance on 'command and control' management prevalent in the NHS. Denning is reminding us (as indeed group analysis has been pointing out for some 50 years) that humans are fundamentally social beings and that we override this at our cost. The need to belong is hard-wired in us, whether described in the language of connection theory, complexity theory, attachment theory or object-relations theory.

The closest I came to experiencing working with Maslow's fourth level goes back to the decade of the 1980s at St George's Hospital. Yet I will admit that our youthful enthusiasm would have died a slow death had we not had the funds to implement our good intentions.

---

15. Denning (2010).

The Fifth Level: Self-actualisation

To illustrate the dynamics on this level, I should explain that Maslow described two contrasting kinds of need. First, there are the needs outlined so far, concerned with safety, nourishment, love, belonging, respect and self-esteem. Maslow called these 'deficiency needs' (D-needs). However, Maslow wanted to give equal weight to psychological well-being. He felt that humanity aspired naturally towards 'being values' (B-values) such as unity, transcendence, aliveness, uniqueness, justice, order, simplicity, goodness and truth. Such values are sustained by B-needs that are expansive, for example, the need to engage in meaningful, helpful work and service, to promote justice and harmony and to express one's creativity. The difference can be illustrated with a single example: the need to be loved is a D-need and the need to love is a B-need.[16]

According to Maslow, self-actualisation includes: accurate perception of reality; comfortable acceptance of self and others; tolerance of human imperfection and the ability to laugh at oneself; living with vitality and spontaneity; being comfortable in solitude; desiring to work for the benefit of humankind; a capacity for autonomy; appreciation of the gift of life; living fully in the moment; enjoying deep personal relationships; and fellowship with humanity. Maslow concludes by describing the 'peak experience', when self-actualisation is crystallised in a feeling of oneness with all that is, accompanied by intense happiness that confirms the value, purpose and meaning of life.

Maslow distinguished two psychological profiles among self-actualisers: 'transcenders', who are drawn to peak experiences, and 'non-transcenders' (who Maslow also called 'healthy self-actualisers'), characterised by their resilience and groundedness. No stereotyping applies here; a businessman may be a transcender and a good priest a non-transcender; Maslow believed that every human being has the potential for self-actualisation in one or other form, and that human society needs both.

Caring for the Carers

How might we work with Maslow's ideas in a modern health service? Firstly, there are basic practical concerns that must be addressed.

---

16. Maslow's D-needs and B-needs correspond closely to the needs of the ego and the needs of the soul respectively, as described elsewhere in this volume.

Beginning with the first level of need, there should be provision for proper rest and sleep, with nourishing food and protected time for eating in comfort away from the clinical environment. This makes a big difference to working long shifts. Calls could be filtered so that only genuine emergencies intrude at these times.

Doctors are often afraid to complain about working hours and conditions in case it damages their career prospects. The European Working Time Directive of 48 hours per week needs to be implemented as it was intended, not averaged out over six-monthly periods. The CQC has identified serious staffing shortages, with major resource implications that would have to be faced.[17]

Maslow's second level of safety is an absolute prerequisite before a workplace can feel secure and welcoming. Trust management needs to address the lack of confidence that doctors have in them. It used to be understood that the doctor's first concern and loyalty was to their patients and that the hospital was there to provide the facilities and the support. If a trust is struggling financially and already feels under threat, doctors working there are likely to feel unsupported when clinical mistakes are made. It is then all the harder to admit to errors of judgement or to whistle-blow.

David Nicholson, CEO of the NHS, announced in 2013 that 400 gagging clauses would be lifted retrospectively, with no further gagging allowed.[18] There is also to be 'duty of candour', a contractual obligation for NHS providers to be transparent over failures of medical and nursing management, a measure intended to redress the lack of trust between patients, their families and care providers when things go wrong.

In order to establish the third level, of belonging and acceptance, peer group support is an important element. For instance, how would it be if consultants – others too – met weekly for lunch, not the notorious 'working lunch', but to share an hour together eating and conversing in peace and quiet? This used to happen before job plans had to account for every minute of the working day. 'Time and motion' mentality may help set targets but is not conducive to goodwill and friendship, and the benefits that derive.

At the fourth level, of esteem and respect, there is a problem for the mental health service, which does not reward with an abundance of grateful patients and therapeutic triumphs. Many mental disorders are enduring and the prevalence of depression, with constant concern

---

17. For a comprehensive update, see Care Quality Commission (2016).
18. Dominiczak (2013).

about patients who may self-harm, can put extreme stress on carers. This burden was once recognised in the form of a favourable early retirement pension option for mental health officers – these days no longer available. Working in front line psychiatry carries the insidious danger of draining joy out of life. There is now a serious recruitment problem, with many staff leaving the NHS to work in private practice or abroad.

The great majority of mental health professionals choose the specialty from a sense of vocation, and at its best, there is no finer act of service. However, if a person is to be open to mental suffering and able to respond with empathy, ongoing support is needed. Trusts and clinical tutors could start by endorsing Balint peer groups,[19] in which staff can share the difficulties they encounter and together explore how their inner resources can be best used to cope and to care.

Behind these suggestions lies an implicit reminder. In the turmoil of daily life, we can easily feel ourselves victims of a persecutory regime that is forcing us with threats and demands to do ever more. Yet it can only happen when we lose sight of our self-sovereignty and forget that we do not actually have to do everything we are told, but instead can decide a great many things for ourselves.

This brings me to self-actualisation, the fifth and final level. Thus far, I have set out the preconditions that Maslow argues are required, and they are compelling. His schema takes us from one level to the next and it all makes good sense. Meeting the needs that Maslow outlines would surely improve well-being and make for better healthcare. However, if we waited for a social revolution to bring about this utopia, we would wait for a lifetime. Fortunately, there are already good people around who have found ways to bring their creativity and compassion to bear – and who inspire us to try to do likewise.

I began by reminiscing about how things used to be. It is worth doing so, because history can spare us from having to re-invent the wheel. However, it does not help to blame anyone or anything for how things are today. To do so would be to suppose things could have or should have turned out differently. This is a fruitless line of enquiry, since if things could have been different, then they would have been!

This suggests that rather than wringing our hands over the parlous state of things, the task is to work at what one can without fear or favour. Doing so is not always easy, since we are all anxious not to lose our reputation, credibility, friendships, jobs, health and more. Nevertheless, we need to find a way to overcome such anxiety if we are

---

19. For a brief summary, see Salinsky (2009).

to keep calm, stay in touch with our humanity and respond to suffering with compassion. Then we can maintain equanimity when success is followed by reversal, or when a good plan dies in committee! We simply continue to do what we can for our patients with love and goodwill.

The ethos of an institution can only be sustained by its workforce. I have drawn on Maslow's hierarchy of needs to illustrate the complex social matrix that comprises the NHS. Given the serious current spending shortfall, there is all the more need to care for its staff, otherwise no amount of 'efficiency savings' or 'rationalisation of resources' will do any good.[20] NHS management urgently needs to understand this. The current obsession with numbers on a page risks de-humanising what is the most human of all vocations – healthcare. Maslow offers a model of care that would serve the NHS well, not only bringing the focus back to the human being, but also leading to best clinical practice. Think what a self-actualised NHS could achieve!

References

Bauby, J-D. (1998) *The Diving Bell and the Butterfly: A Memoir of Life in Death*. Vintage Books.

BBC One (2011) Panorama: 'Undercover care: the abuse exposed'. BBC. Available at: http://documentaryheaven.com/undercover-care/ (accessed 7 July 2017).

Campbell, D. (2013) Jeremy Hunt: NHS errors mean eight patients die a day. *The Guardian*, 21 June. Available at: http://www.theguardian.com/politics/2013/jun/21/jeremy-hunt-nhs-errors-patients (accessed 7 July 2017).

Care Quality Commission (2011) *Dignity and Nutrition Inspection Programme: National Overview*. CQC. Available at: http://www.cqc.org.uk/sites/default/files/documents/20111007_dignity_and_nutrition_inspection_report_final_update.pdf (accessed 7 July 2017).

Care Quality Commission (2016) *The State of Care in NHS Acute Hospitals: 2014 to 2016*. CQC. Available at: http://www.cqc.org.uk/sites/default/files/20170302b_stateofhospitals_web.pdf (accessed 12 July 2017).

Denning, S. (2010) *The Leader's Guide to Radical Management: Reinventing the Workplace for the 21st Century*. Jossey-Bass.

Department of Health (2012) *Transforming Care: A National Response to Winterbourne View Hospital (Department of Health Review – Final Report)*. Department of Health. Available at: https://www.gov.uk/government/uploads/system/uploads/attachment_data/file/213216/easy-read-of-final-report.pdf (accessed 7 July 2017).

---

20. When this paper was written, there was hope of an economic upturn that would relieve some of the financial pressures on the NHS. Far from happening, there has been a continuing economic downturn and consequently the crisis facing the NHS in 2017 is greater than at any other time.

Dominiczak, P. (2013) Gagged NHS whistleblowers will be allowed to speak out, Sir David Nicholson says. *The Telegraph*, 18 March. Available at: http://www.telegraph.co.uk/news/uknews/9938809/Gagged-NHS-whistleblowers-will-be-allowed-to-speak-out-Sir-David-Nicholson-says.html (accessed 7 July 2017).

Francis, R. (2013) *Report of the Mid Staffordshire NHS Foundation Trust Public Inquiry (The Francis Report)*. Available at: www.midstaffspublicinquiry.com (accessed 7 July 2017).

Lampard, K. & Marsden, E. (2015) *Themes and Lessons Learnt from NHS Investigations into Matters Relating to Jimmy Savile. Independent Report for the Secretary of State for Health*. Department of Health. Available at: https://www.gov.uk/government/publications/jimmy-savile-nhs-investigations-lessons-learned (accessed 7 July 2017).

Lorrance, A. (2001) *The Love Principles*. Wisdom Books.

Maslow, A. (1943) A theory of human motivation. *Psychological Review*, 50, 370–396.

Mental Health Foundation (2016) Mental Health and Prevention: Taking Local Action for Better Mental Health. Mental Health Foundation. Available at: https://www.mentalhealth.org.uk/publications/mental-health-and-prevention-taking-local-action-better-mental-health (accessed 7 July 2017).

Pierce, A. (2013) NHS spends £15million (the same as 750 nurses' salaries) on gagging 600 whistleblowers. *Mail Online*, 22 February. Available at: http://www.dailymail.co.uk/news/article-2282600/NHS-spends-15million-750-nurses-salaries-gagging-600-whistleblowers.html (accessed 7 July 2017).

Salinsky, J. (2009) A very short introduction to Balint groups. The Balint Society. Available at: http://balint.co.uk/about/introduction/ (accessed 7 July 2017).

11

The Whole Patient

By the word 'whole' I mean to convey 'the full quantity, amount, extent, without diminution or exception, undivided, a unity, entire, and complete in itself'.[1]

Pictorial images of wholeness are found throughout history in the form of *mandalas* – mandala being Sanskrit for circle. In Hinduism and Buddhism, these sacred images symbolise the whole universe depicted as a microcosm. In a similar vein, there is the age-old description of the Divine as an infinite sphere, whose centre is everywhere and whose circumference is nowhere.[2] It may be no coincidence that from a very different quarter, cosmologists have now discovered that this turns out to be an apt conceptualisation of the universe.[3]

In this discussion of wholeness, I shall be treating the physical and the metaphysical worlds as two sides of one coin and so I shall be speaking of body and soul, although I am well aware that 'soul' is not a word often heard on a hospital ward.

Wholeness and the Discovery of Selfhood

Much of life is concerned with surviving traumas that threaten a person's sense of wholeness. Very likely this is why we are attracted to the wholeness that we sense in the innocent being of a happy baby, stirring trace memories of our own brief sojourn in that Garden of Eden.

Paper prepared for the Well-being, Health and Wholeness Forum, London, April 2013.

---

1. The Concise Oxford Dictionary of Current English (8th edition).
2. Variously attributed to the philosopher Empedocles (5th century BCE), the grammarian and philosopher Marius Victorinus (4th century CE) or the mythical figure of Hermes Trismegistus. Later enshrined in the writings of Cardinal Nicolas of Cusa (15th century CE).
3. For a detailed account, see Teerikorpi (2009).

Babies are not yet self-aware, since to begin with there is no perceptual delimitation of the self. At around 18 months, a toddler will look into a mirror and grasp that the reflection is of their own bodily self. There follows the realisation of a divide between self and world, one that bestows the privacy of an inner existence – along with new independence of mind. Yet in discovering that the self is bounded, the child is obliged to face that they are alone – a leitmotif that weaves its way through the history of human consciousness.

If we have been loved and cherished early in life, we internalise good parental imagos that we can draw on when needed as an inner source of comfort and love – in effect, learning how to parent ourselves. In this way, a child can sustain a sense of wholeness while exploring the wider world. However, when something goes wrong and the child is distressed, the sense of wholeness is under threat and can rapidly fall apart unless a loving caregiver is there to step in and help restore confidence.

As we continue to grow and become more competent at survival, we learn the complex rules of life – when to observe them, when to bend them and when sometimes to break them. At the same time, we acquire a variety of roles intrinsic to our maturing sense of identity, as worker, friend, lover, spouse, parent and more. Throughout the first half of life, during what has been called the outward journey, a great deal of energy goes into fulfilling those roles as best we can. For this, we depend on the ego, with its hopes, fears, drives and defences that enable us to steer a course through life. Yet for everyone the day must come when the 'return journey' begins. It may be occasioned by illness, loss, emotional trauma or simply when a person otherwise in good health suddenly notices how life is slipping by them. At any rate, whether it comes sooner or later, we are challenged to take stock of the whole shape of our lives – what has been, what is, and what remains. Not least, the fond illusion of immortality recedes as we begin to face the ending that must come. This realisation also brings the opportunity to find out that beyond the many roles of personhood there is another, deeper layer to the self, a centre of stillness that transcends the helter-skelter of emotions that dominate so much of life. This is the dwelling place of the soul, from where it is possible to view life and the drama of human affairs with equanimity, tolerance and lightness of being.

The soul was, in its essence, always there. It can be first seen, remarkably, in the eyes of the newborn[4] and in the clear and trusting

---

4. See also *The Soul of the Newborn Child*, in Powell (2017).

gaze of a child. Year on year, the soul quietly accompanies the ego in its worldly travails, patiently encouraging it to progress from preoccupation with itself to caring for others – in other words, from learning how to survive to learning how to love.

Wholeness and the Impact of Illness

It has been rather shockingly remarked that life is a sexually transmitted disease for which there is no treatment and which is uniformly fatal! The human ego cannot bear this grim fact, since it is dedicated to being strong and well, overcoming illness or disability, being potent in every sense and achieving great things. This means rejecting any intimation of mortality. Yet, excepting sudden death, we shall, sooner or later and without exception, fall ill and become someone's patient.

I recall two brief but memorable episodes of illness in childhood. When I was ten years old and at my boarding preparatory school, I developed an acute ear infection. It was treated cursorily by the school matron, who did not hide her contempt for me, since I was habitually homesick. The pain in my ear was agonising, made worse because I felt I was not believed. Fortunately, the school term was just ending and as soon as I arrived home, my mother rushed me to the local hospital, where a kindly doctor examined me. I remember the hiss of breath through his teeth as he observed that my eardrum was about to perforate. I was immediately given an injection of penicillin and within twenty-four hours, I had recovered.

The second time, I was twelve and home on half-term exeat. I woke with a tummy-ache, which by the next day was much worse. Our family doctor arranged for a domiciliary visit by a surgeon, who felt my tummy, admitted me to hospital on the spot and removed my appendix the same day.

I am sure these events played their part in my wanting to become a doctor, just as I have no doubt that the unhappiness of those long years away at school influenced my choosing later to specialise in psychiatry.

Short-lived illnesses of one sort or another affect us all at some time. We are stoical, complaining, made anxious or treat them with bravado according to our disposition and cultural conditioning. Sympathy and support from loved ones and friends, and the right medical help, usually get us through unscathed so that the problem of wholeness, or rather the lack of it, is short-lived.

When illnesses are more complex and enduring, the defences employed by the ego to shield the self from anxiety, often by means of denial, can be powerfully activated, sometimes at great personal cost. I remember examining a woman with advanced breast cancer, who only came for help when her breasts were so swollen she could no longer find a bra to fit. There was a man facing potential amputation of his legs due to vascular disease, who refused to admit that his continuing heavy smoking had anything to do with his blocked femoral arteries. The moment the consultant left, the patient wheeled himself out of the ward to get another smoke.

Denial is not exclusive to our patients. Doctors can suffer from it too, especially when we attempt to treat at all costs – hence the quip 'the treatment worked but the patient died'. I recall a visibly frail man who had a series of cardiac arrests in the coronary care unit, where I was working as a young doctor. Each time we defibrillated him he regained consciousness, and then a few hours later there would be another arrest. After the fourth time, as I was leaning over him, he whispered 'Let me go'. I was so determined to win the day I did not, or could not, heed what he was saying. The next time his heart stopped, it resisted all of our heroic efforts. It was a lesson I have never forgotten – that our patients sometimes know what is best for them.

Whole Patient, Whole Doctor

Patient and doctor are in complementary roles, since there would be no doctors without patients and *vice versa*. As every medical student quickly learns, few people are concise and clear historians. The doctor must lead, guide and maintain clarity, a clinical skill that calls for empathy as well as medical acumen.

When a patient senses that his or her distress is being responded to with understanding, the barriers come down, ego defences are set aside and the natural anxiety that goes with falling ill can be allowed to speak. Illness brings out the child in us. It is an understandable, temporary regression which, when handled appropriately, helps us manage our fears. In the parlance of psychoanalysis, a good doctor meets the transference need of the patient – to be cared for by a trusted parent figure who will put right what is wrong and so, hopefully, restore the patient to health.

The Constitution of the World Health Organization (WHO) defines health as 'a state of complete physical, mental and social well-being and not merely the absence of disease'.[5] In another publication, it goes on to say:

> '...the health professions have largely followed a medical model, which seeks to treat patients by focusing on medicines and surgery, and gives less importance to beliefs and faith (in healing, in the physician and in the doctor-patient relationship). This reductionism or mechanistic view of patients as being only a material body, is no longer satisfactory. Patients and physicians have begun to realise the value of elements such as faith, hope and compassion in the healing process.'[6]

This statement is timely and important, yet the context also needs taking into account. When I had acute appendicitis, I did not need a lengthy heart-to-heart with the surgeon. He was brisk, friendly, said what was needed, did his job and was gone. It was entirely different when as a young doctor, my family and I had to face that our newborn would only be with us for a short while. The consultant paediatrician, a kindly, unassuming man, knew how to listen and most importantly, never seemed to be in a hurry. We took comfort from his wholeness of presence, natural humility and compassion, while we awaited an outcome that was to be inevitable and final.

Any discussion of wholeness means looking through more than one lens. To begin with, there is the naive wholeness that is one's healthy biological endowment and that most people enjoy unthinkingly. The life force is strong; *mens sana in corpore sano* – sound mind in sound body. An unforeseen illness briefly knocks us over, but we bounce back – whole again! The vagaries of the human condition will inevitably test us but mostly we do not, thank goodness, succumb.

Then there are illnesses that affect us more deeply. I related two from my childhood that stand out because the dramatic interventions of those two doctors exerted an influence on my life greater than I could have foreseen. Serious illness is life changing, having the potential to diminish or enhance us according to what we make of the experience. When I was fifty, I underwent heart surgery, which was followed by pneumonia. I found out what it was like to be unable to think straight or take a decent breath and getting in and out of bed was tantamount to climbing a mountain. I slowly recovered, became ambulant and began

---

5. Preamble to the Constitution of WHO as adopted by the International Health Conference, New York, 19 June – 22 July 1946; signed on 22 July 1946 by the representatives of 61 States (Official Records of WHO, no. 2, p. 100) and entered into force on 7 April 1948.
6. World Health Organization (1998: 7). Also referenced in *Whither the Soul of Psychiatry?*, this volume.

to retrieve my mind. My new lease of life brought home to me in a very personal way that firstly, to enjoy clarity of consciousness is nothing short of a miracle and that secondly, we need love in order to heal.

There was a remarkable interview on television during the Paralympic Games of 2012, when an amputee who had just received a gold medal was asked if she wished she could have her limb back. She declared unhesitatingly, 'No, because then I would never have had this moment'. What had started as a devastating blow to the ego had become the emblem of her triumph over loss. She had found wholeness, perhaps more so than she had ever known before.

This underlines that wholeness is a way of being, not merely the impression made by physicality. At the age of 40, the renowned psychodramatist Zerka Moreno was diagnosed with sarcoma of the right arm and was advised that her arm and shoulder should be amputated. Unable to bear the prospect of such disfiguring surgery, she turned to psychodrama for help. In her hospital room, Zerka first asked God whether she should have the operation. Then, reversing roles with God, Zerka found herself (as God) answering with serene authority, 'The choice is yours. You can keep your arm but you *will* die, or you can lose it and live'.[7] Subsequently, on first meeting Zerka, people would often fail to notice that her arm was missing, such was her wholeness of being.

Mental Illness and Afflictions of the Soul

Disorders of mental health are invariably complex and life changing, since mental illness, whatever the cause, is indicative of a fractured self. Furthermore, mental illness in high-income societies is now on an epidemic scale.[8]

Is the human race suffering from some kind of biological meltdown or are we in the grip of a malaise that has taken hold of human society? Could it be that living in a post-modern world, where cost comes first and value second, great numbers of people are afflicted with problems of identity, meaning and purpose? It seems to me that in the 21st century, we appear to be heading away from, rather than towards, a healthier, happier world.

What is the hard-pressed doctor supposed to do? Most doctors are not by nature social visionaries, political activists or aiming to be

---

7. Personal communication (1976).
8. For more detailed epidemiological data, see *Recovery and Well-Being: The Search for the Soul* and *Helping Patients Tell Their Story: Narratives of Body, Mind and Soul*, both this volume.

senior managers of the service. They just want to get on with seeing their patients in the customary way and to diagnose and treat so far as the pragmatics of healthcare will allow.

There is a common subjective end-point to all suffering – a loss of wholeness that results in a person feeling estranged from both themselves and others. One way to help is to overcome this estrangement by ensuring that the relationship between practitioner and patient is authentic, trustworthy and compassionate. This is the medicine of the soul, and while it may not be the only medicine required, it should be the first to be offered. The way is then open to explore whether the symptom may be indicative of the need to make life changes that would benefit the patient's health and well-being.

What Do We Mean by Soul?

There can be no one definition of the soul,[9] since its numinous quality evokes a meaning that is personal to the individual. Nonetheless, most people find the word holds for them a deep resonance. Some take the secular viewpoint that it simply symbolises the finest values and aspirations of humankind. For others, the soul conjures up the most profound experience of what it means 'to be' – a state of calm and peace when the noisy chatter of the mind is stilled. Many believe the soul to be non-corporeal yet as 'real' as the physical body, being a scintilla of the Divine present in every human being. Going still further, there are those who hold that the soul incarnates in order to give of itself to humanity, to experience life through human eyes and to take all it has learned with it when it leaves.

While I happen to subscribe to all these views (for they are not exclusive), what I want to highlight here is that the soul is profoundly subjective, that it lives fully in the 'now' and is deeply engaged in the human journey while knowing and understanding that 'all things must pass'.[10]

Most importantly, the soul simply loves to 'be'. Because this exuberance of love flows from the same wellspring for all humanity, the soul sees all selves as reflections of the one self. This is the basis of the 'golden rule' found in the precepts of every spiritual and religious tradition – that in what we do to others, we are doing the same to ourselves.

---

9. Also discussed in *Recovery and Well-Being*, this volume.
10. For the purpose of this discussion, it makes no difference which view of the soul a doctor holds. Provided there is sensitivity to, and genuine respect for, the patient's beliefs, the relationship will be experienced as life enhancing, not least in the face of serious illness.

The Soul of Medicine

Medicine as a vocation was never born of reason; it arises from the natural impulse of the soul and we are not required to be spiritual masters to converse soul to soul with our patients. I am suggesting that the soul will make its presence felt provided that the ego, with its many agendas based on conditionality, can be set aside for a while. Then empathy arises, and kindness, too. The doctor/patient relationship is uniquely privileged, for when a soul connection is made, no matter how grave the situation, the patient will feel heartened.[11]

There is no prescribed content to soul talk; it could happen in a split second in the appreciation of flowers on a bedside table, the touch of a hand, sharing good news or breaking bad news. Whatever arises will happen naturally and exactly as it should when the doctor is able to be fully 'present', unafraid, genuinely open to what their patient is experiencing and helping find the way forward that is in the patient's best interests.

Wholeness at the End of Life

When a person is suffering from terminal illness, doctors may experience helplessness and a sense of failure. Patients are acutely sensitive to this and we know that in such cases they will try to hide their own anxieties and concerns from their doctor. Yet hospices specialising in end-of-life care have shown that this can be a very special time; pretences and evasions can be relinquished and there is a precious opportunity for reconciliation and forgiveness, not only with others but also with the self. Enabling the soul to find expression heals the splits in the psyche that we all incur during our lifetime. There need be no shame, for the soul embraces the bruised and battered ego with the same unconditional welcome that greeted the return of the prodigal son.[12]

Helping one's patient to die with a sense of wholeness means to enable a person to die healed. This is not the contradiction that it might appear to be. The human journey that began with wholeness should, whenever possible, end with wholeness. In between, where we do our living, suffering, separation and loss are inevitable.[13] Yet thanks

---

11. The essence of good doctoring: 'Every time a doctor sees a patient, the patient should feel better as a result'. In Lown (1996: 88).
12. The parable of the lost son, in which love forgives all. Luke 15:11–32. *The Holy Bible*, NIV.
13. Hence the saying, 'God never promises a smooth crossing; only a safe landing'.

to the soul, the Garden of Eden from whence we came is never lost to us, even though we may no longer consciously remember our innocent beginnings. With the passing of the years, we become aware that the epic drama of the ego is a play on which the curtain must fall. Watching the many scenes of one's life from the vantage of protagonist, playwright, director and audience (for the soul sees all), the oneness that underlies all of life is revealed once again, so that 'the full quantity, amount, extent, without diminution or exception, undivided, a unity, entire, and complete in itself' is restored.

References

Lown, B. (1996) *The Lost Art of Healing: Practicing Compassion in Medicine*. Random House.
Powell, A. (2017) *The Ways of the Soul. A Psychiatrist Reflects: Essays on Life, Death and Beyond*. Muswell Hill Press.
Teerikorpi, P. (2009) *The Evolving Universe and the Origin of Life: The Search for Our Cosmic Roots*. Springer.
World Health Organization (1998) *WHOQOL and Spirituality, Religiousness and Personal Beliefs (SRPB): Report on WHO Consultation*. WHO. Available at: http://apps.who.int/iris/handle/10665/70897 (accessed 8 July 2017).

12

What Does It Mean to be Human?

All of life is contained in the question 'What does it mean to be human?', since everything we know about our existence is either apperceived by means of our sense organs or conceptualised by the human mind. Indeed, what does it mean to be *not* human? We can only guess!

We cannot discuss our human need to make sense of and give purpose to our lives without taking into proper account that we are conscious beings, a faculty we share with many sentient life forms. Furthermore, *Homo sapiens* is a bio-socio-psycho-spiritual being and so the question applies to all these aspects of humanity.

On the biological level, the human species is the most complex and advanced life form on the planet, a biped whose evolutionary prowess has bestowed immense power both to create and to destroy. We are a very recent species. Fossil remains of *Homo habilis*, along with their early stone tools, go back a mere couple of million years, followed by *Homo erectus* around 1 million years ago, and then *Homo sapiens* some half a million years later. A massive enlargement of the neocortex, comprising the frontal lobes of the brain, has resulted in exceptional intelligence and most importantly, self-awareness, a crucial development I will refer to again.

On the societal level, we live in a highly complex world of relationships. Care of the young provides protective and nurturing characteristics similar to those in other higher mammalian species and there is a lengthy process of cognitive and emotional maturation until myelination of the brain has been fully completed in adulthood. Human society is still largely territorial (based on ethnicity, nationality, culture and religion), but elaborated emotionally and intellectually by the human capacity for language, thought and symbolisation. This has resulted in a rich, creative and artistic cultural history.

Preface to 'What Does It Mean to be Human?', a dialogue with the Revd Christopher MacKenna, held by the Guild of Pastoral Psychology, London, May 2013.

Through the power to manipulate the environment, science and technology have brought immense benefits to what we call the civilised world in terms of human welfare, health, comfort and longevity. However, given the times in which we are now living, the negative side of technological prowess has to be acknowledged. Our species, still in the kindergarten of its evolution, enacts aggression on a global scale, having killed over 130 million of its own kind in the 20th century – more than throughout all the previous time-line of history. Indeed, we might as well be called *Homo ignorans*, for in a collective assault on the delicate ecosystems of the natural world, it is just possible we will bring about our own extinction in the next hundred years, if not sooner.

On the psychological level, we exhibit a strange mix of thoughtful insight and chaotic emotion. This has brought about a great deal of suffering to date – a cardinal feature of the human condition. Suffering is the reaction to loss, real, threatened or fantasied, including foreknowledge of one's own inevitable death. Nonetheless, the poignant nature of loss has been a profound spur to the cultural history of humanity in painting, literature and music.

On the spiritual level, East and West have held rather different attitudes to suffering. In the East, it is treated stoically as something to overcome by detachment of the ego, as in Buddhism and Daoism. In the West, with roots in the Abrahamic faith traditions, suffering is more often taken to be the path to redemption and salvation. All spirituality, however, works towards the same end – that of an evolved psyche, bringing a more expansive, loving and unitary view of life.

Also on the spiritual level, we can appreciate both the strengths and limitations of the human ego. The ego's crowning achievement has been self-awareness. On the one hand, self-awareness profoundly separates us from the unitive consciousness that undergirds all of life. Unfortunately, this can lead to the folly of supposing we humans know better than Nature. On the other hand, without the ego there would be no duality of subject and object and thus no capacity for self-reflection, insight or learning, neither the many hues of feeling that enrich life.

The ego needs the guidance of wisdom if it is to be harnessed for the betterment of humankind. Wisdom arises when experience is comprehended with love, as we discover when we are attuned to the soul. Along with myriad sentient life forms – for the universe is vast – I like to think that we are thereby enabling God to get to know more of God. Not least, if humanity wakes up to the realisation that the foundation of all life is the one life, we have a great opportunity to stop hurting each other and start making Heaven on Earth.

Science has traditionally been the adversary of religion. This goes back to the mechanistic interpretation of Newtonian physics that sees humankind as nothing but a chance biological life form existing in an otherwise largely lifeless universe. Yet the classical physics of material realism is being challenged by a new cosmology, born of quantum physics, that transcends the limits of space-time. Consciousness, for so long disregarded by science, is centre-stage in this new, participative cosmology. The human ego might feel both flattered and humbled if we discovered that inasmuch as the universe conjures us into existence, we conjure it into being with our consciousness. I say 'our' consciousness but in all likelihood, there is but one consciousness, and just as the buds that flower on a tree have no choice in the matter, we take our place in the greater design of things. It is wonderful that we can know this, witness it, and thereby celebrate both our humanity and our divinity.

13

The Place of Medicine in Today's World

I qualified as a doctor in 1969. Technology has since changed the face of medicine. In those days, a few daring surgeons were replacing heart valves, usually on patients in extremis. These days, such procedures are routine and I happen to be one of the many beneficiaries. At the same time, there are huge problems with the delivery of person-centred healthcare, due in part to the super-specialisation that accompanies a multitude of technical advances.

While more fortunate individuals benefit from sophisticated interventions, healthcare on a global scale nevertheless faces unprecedented challenges. To examine this further, we need to step outside the familiar setting of the consulting room and take a look at what is going on in the wider world.

The problem can be compared with the dilemma that besets a good many parents whose egalitarian ideals favour universal state-funded education, but who end up paying for private schooling in order to give their children what they hope will be the best start in life. For example, the aortic valve prosthesis that spared me an early grave could be seen as an indefensible privilege when one looks at the scale of disease decimating the human population in many parts of the world. A great deal of medical research is geared to the treatment of conditions only affordable to the more economically developed countries. As it happens, citizens of these countries are generally the costliest to treat because so many of their ailments are self-inflicted: the prevalence of diabetes linked with obesity, the 50% lifetime risk of cancer associated with increased longevity, the soaring incidence of cardiovascular disease arising from a stressful and sedentary lifestyle and the morbidity associated with alcohol, drugs and tobacco consumption, to name but a few.

Paper prepared for the Scientific and Medical Network Round Table Conference 'Transforming Worldviews in Science, Medicine and Psychology', Horsham, July 2013.

Investment in cutting-edge technology is no longer confined to the Western world. For around 3000 years, China relied on classical Chinese medicine, using herbal treatments, acupuncture and medical Qigong to supplement a lifestyle of moderation and balance based on Daoist principles of healthcare.[1] There is a folk saying in China, 'Calling for the doctor when you are ill is like having to dig a well when you are thirsty!' However, the tradition of preventative medicine in China is rapidly being supplanted by Westernisation of diet, lifestyle and high-tech medical intervention.

Today, the practice of modern medicine highlights a real dilemma for humanity. Of course, we physicians wish to help our fellow human beings with all the skills at our disposal. The root of the word medicine comes from the Latin verb *mederi*, which is 'to heal'. The noun *medicina* means 'the art of healing'. This goes hand in hand with Hippocrates' counsel: 'Cure sometimes, treat often, comfort always', very much directed at the needs of the whole person.

Western medicine, however, is rooted deep in the soil of reductionism, a movement that began during the Renaissance with the dissection of the human cadaver. The identification of organ function followed, and hence our mechanistic understanding of the human body, which to this day focusses on the part rather than the whole.[2]

From an archetypal perspective, Western medicine is a triumph of the analytical masculine mind. The problem lies in having devalued the feminine principle, which knows the whole to be greater than the sum of the parts, whether speaking of humanity or the natural world. Yet I am not reproaching the medical profession, for mainstream healthcare is a social institution and is simply mirroring the mindset of society. If humankind could grasp the meaning of the whole, it could not behave in the wanton way it does, despoiling the planet and killing large numbers of its own kind. (I have wondered if testosterone should carry a health warning, for no sooner than it brings life to the womb, it dispatches it on the battlefield.)

We know that the greatest benefits to the health of a given population come through the right kind of diet, exercise, good housing, effective sanitation, sobriety and responsible sexual behaviour. Add to this the proper management of childbirth and vaccination against the principal infectious diseases and, from the perspective of the species, humanity would have been well served. The natural lifespan would

---

1. Guo & Powell (2001).
2. Neuroscience similarly adheres to this tradition in seeking to reduce the human mind to the physical substratum of the brain.

have been reasonably extended, and were it to be coupled with an agreed limit on family size to, say, two children, the problem of caring for an increasing geriatric population with its complex care needs would be solved.

If we could only stop there! But of course, we can't and don't. What is happening is unstoppable, for humanity is set on a course driven more by intellect than wisdom and enchanted by technologies that excite rather than caution. As a result, in a mere couple of hundred years, human beings have put a large question mark against the survival of our species, indeed all species that depend on the fragile ecosystems of this planet.

The science of medicine is inextricably bound to the achievements and ambitions of modernity, which at best has pioneered life-saving prostheses like heart valves, yet which, at the same time, makes and sells junk foods that clog the arterial tree. At its best, medicine has saved countless lives with the help of antibiotics. Yet, due to their profligate misuse, we now have bacteria that are resistant to every known antibiotic and which will soon return us to the days of Joseph Lister[3] and antisepsis. At best, thanks to Edward Jenner's historic researches,[4] we have eliminated smallpox. Yet in 2010, the avian and human flu viruses were genetically combined with a potential for human-to-human transmission.[5] (We are told there is no danger since the hybrid virus is safely secured in a bio-lab!) At best, we can perform liver transplants and yet we make billions from the sale of the alcohol that causes cirrhosis. At best, we can vaccinate against the sexually transmitted human papilloma virus that causes cancer of the cervix. Yet we now live with an epidemic of HIV due to a culture of sexual promiscuity.

In the field of mental health, which has been my specialty, severe mental illness, namely bipolar disorder and schizophrenia, continue to have prevalence of 1–2% each, regardless of nationality, culture or ethnicity. We still do not understand the causes and while symptoms

---

3. Joseph Lister (1827–1912), later 1st Baron Lister, was the first surgeon to apply Louis Pasteur's findings in microbiology, carrying out operations under sterile conditions using antisepsis (carbolic acid) and thereby drastically reducing wound infection, the major cause of all postoperative deaths.
4. Edward Jenner (1749–1823) developed immunisation against smallpox by inoculation with the cowpox virus. Smallpox, from which over 2 million died as late as 1969, was declared globally eradicated by the World Health Organization in 1979.
5. Research programme funded and jointly carried out by the US National Institutes of Health, the Japan Society for the Promotion of Science and the Japan Science and Technology Agency.

may respond to medication, cure remains a distant hope. In addition, psychiatrists and general practitioners are expected to treat a social epidemic of human misery now labelled depression – one that works greatly to the advantage of the pharmaceutical industry. Why so much unhappiness? Perhaps because consumerism, material realism and the breakdown of traditional values in the post-modern world have exacerbated a culture of anomie first described by Emile Durkheim over a hundred years ago.

In today's world, we are living with a grievous loss of soul, both individually and collectively. Yet much of mainstream psychiatry, shaped by the culture of science, is concerned primarily with things that can be measured. In the Spirituality and Psychiatry Special Interest Group of the Royal College of Psychiatrists[6] we do our best to redress the imbalance. We know the interest in spirituality is there, for one in six UK psychiatrists are members of the group. Yet apart from mindfulness-based cognitive therapy and some programmes for the treatment of substance misuse, spiritually informed treatments are not generally available within the National Health Service.[7] Such therapies (like most of complementary medicine) have to be sought in the private sector, which relies on individual recommendation rather than on evidence-based medicine.

Over the past 50 years, medical science has accomplished many wonderful things, not least thanks to advances in technology. Unfortunately, by the same token, we are in danger of losing the human face of medicine. To use a well-worn metaphor, our fascination with the car may lead us to forget the driver.

Should we be surprised that this is happening? When we mistake the part for the whole, we lose the capacity to see beyond the playground of the ego, a world of dualities in which even the brightest light cannot banish the shadow. Is it so strange that the scourges of the Middle Ages, smallpox, leprosy, bubonic plague, are being replaced today with drug-resistant tuberculosis, malaria, and HIV? We fight disease with everything to hand but it keeps coming back![8]

It is only natural to wish to avoid physical and mental suffering, to hope for a good life and one that ends with a good death. Individually

---

6. See http://www.rcpsych.ac.uk/spirit
7. Mindfulness is now recommended by the National Institute for Health and Care Excellence (NICE) for the prevention of depression in people who have had three or more bouts of depression in the past. See Crane & Kukyen (2013).
8. Epidemiologists have warned us that unrestricted air travel coupled with growing urban conurbations make the prospect of a devastating influenza pandemic a case of 'not if but when'.

we endeavour to accomplish as much, and medicine, practised well, can certainly help. Yet the destructive aspect of the human ego continues to play havoc with the fate of humankind, leaving charities like Medecins Sans Frontières to pick up the pieces as best they can, in one war zone after another.

People generally view the suffering of humanity as an evil to be overcome on the way to a brighter future. Activists of all persuasions, outraged by the abuses that permeate society, give heart and soul trying to make the world a better place. The problem is that while there are those who care for others, there are others who do not. Each person follows their star for good or ill.

What is to be done? When heartfelt love arises, it does so not because there is an enemy to be defeated (indeed, to do battle is to enlist in a war that never ends). The kind of love the world needs comes from a quickening of the soul. This love is beyond duality, for it takes as axiomatic that *all life is one*. When we stand within that light, indeed when we are one with that light, there is no shadow cast.

Humankind will only emanate that light when we have learned to raise our level of soul consciousness.[9] If we survive long enough as a species, evolution may yet confer the advantage. Meanwhile, we live with the shadow aspect of the human psyche and help as best we can to alleviate the anguish and pain that is visited on humanity. In these circumstances, the physician serves with compassion, restores life when possible and if that cannot be, helps ease our passage when the little wave that is each person's life subsides into the ocean from whence it came.

I, like so many others, am indebted to the profession of medicine for the chance given to the small wave that has been my life to continue a while longer. And when the wave is spent, I shall hope that my doctor, if one should be in attendance, has the wisdom to treat death with the same reverence as life.

References

Crane, R. & Kukyen, W. (2013) The implementation of mindfulness-based cognitive therapy: learning from the UK health service experience. *Mindfulness*, 4, 246–254.
Guo, B. & Powell, A. (2001) *Listen to Your Body – The Wisdom of the Dao*. University of Hawaii Press.

---

9. For a humanistic initiative, see UNESCO (2013). For a contrasting transpersonal initiative, see The Global Consciousness Project (http://noetic.org/research/projects/global-consciousness-project).

UNESCO (2013) Global Consciousness – A Roadmap on Global Consciousness: Thinking and Learning for the 21st Century. UNESCO. Available at: https://en.unesco.org/cultureofpeace/flagship-programmes/global-consciousness (accessed 8 July 2017).

14

Technology and Soul in the 21st Century

In this paper, I shall be exploring the impact of the physical sciences on life, society and the environment, and especially on the young mind. Since I am particularly interested in the perspective of the soul, I will need to begin by saying something about the difference between scientific and spiritual realities.

Science and Spirituality

Science addresses material reality, the physical world of the five senses. It enquires into what things are made of, how things happen, and the way things interact. Science claims to be free of the cultural prejudices that shape our social world, being driven instead by a single imperative – to discover and communicate the impartial truth as revealed by the scientific method.

Science has told us much about the workings of the universe, both within the range of our sense perception and beyond – first X-rays and now the whole field of particle physics. The scientific world-view can be compared with building a house from the various materials brought on site. This is the 'bottom-up' approach, known as upward causation; the bricks are made, as it were, from subatomic particles that stick together and have evolved over billions of years into complex molecules that form the physical universe and everything it contains. The house never needed architect's drawings; it self-assembled.

Since the only reality that science traditionally acknowledges is derived from the five senses, according to classical Newtonian physics, the universe is viewed as a complex mechanical system composed of solid objects, from very small things like microbes to very large things

Paper prepared for keynote talk at the 'Interfaces' event series, Edinburgh International Festival, August 2013.

like planets, separated by air, water, or space – a cosmos that has no purpose or ultimate meaning but is simply there. Most scientists hold that talk of a spiritual world, or of the soul, is a mere product of the imagination. If you cannot measure it, it does not meaningfully exist.[1]

We might have hoped that scientists, with their commitment to rationality, would not suffer from prejudice, but unfortunately the nature of the ego has always been to identify with its own pursuits. People become convinced that they are holding not a belief but the truth and do not like being challenged. In the history of religion, too, radical thinkers were branded heretics. Similarly, in our own time, paranormal research that cannot be explained by the current laws of physics is dismissed by leading science journals on the grounds that the findings are 'impossible'. Such attitudes within science illustrate that the ego is rooted in turf warfare and is ever ready to take offence as much over concepts and beliefs as the defence of one's country, hearth and home.[2]

In contrast to the scientific world-view, spiritual traditions have a 'top-down' approach. Bricks are still needed, but the whole house, so to speak, is born from the potentiality of the supreme consciousness called God (or whichever description is preferred). Why, then, should houses, and people like us who live in them, manifest in this space-time domain? Meister Eckhart, the 13th-century theologian and mystic, answered it this way: 'We are all meant to be mothers of God… for God is always needing to be born'.[3]

The top-down premise cannot be disproven, for there can be no proof that something does not exist. However, the current physicalist narrative of science that dominates contemporary culture has imposed a straightjacket on thinking, all the worse for exercising a prejudice of which people are largely unaware.[4]

Nevertheless, one branch of psychology has been investigating a range of phenomena that challenge physicalism, namely, transpersonal psychology, which has been systematically undertaking research into near-death experiences, out-of-body experiences and after-death communications. The findings suggest that consciousness exists

---

1. This is why consciousness continues to be a thorn in the side of science, which historically has dealt with the problem by ignoring it.
2. Albert Einstein is quoted as having once said that the intuitive mind is a sacred gift and the rational mind is a faithful servant. Remarking on this aphorism, the scholar and visionary Bob Samples observed, 'It is paradoxical that in the context of modern life we have begun to worship the servant and defile the divine'. Samples (1976: 26).
3. Gardner (2016: 35).
4. Physicalism, also known as material realism, holds that everything that exists is based on its physical properties.

independently of physical matter as we know it, something long ruled out of court by conventional physics.[5]

This research coincides with a new explanatory paradigm emerging from advances in quantum mechanics and cosmology that supersedes the billiard ball picture of stars and planets suspended in empty space. We now know that only 5% of the universe is accessed by our senses. The other 95%, of dark matter and dark energy, comprises a single field that is thought to be infinite and timeless, in which, according to the quantum physicist David Bohm, every point in the universe is connected to every other point, forming 'one unbroken whole'.[6]

Holograms reveal this underlying unity. A laser beam, shone on photographic plate imprinted with an interference pattern, will continue to generate the same picture of, say, a three-dimensional apple, whether the photographic plate is cut in two, ten or twenty pieces. Each piece produces the same image, although the smaller the piece, the fuzzier the image. Even so, the image of the whole apple always appears, for no matter how small, the part still contains the whole. Studies of fractals demonstrate the same 'Russian doll' effect. Magnify the edge of a snowflake and it is found to be composed of myriad smaller flakes of the same pattern. Such patterns are replicated over and over, from the very large to the very small, suggesting that the universe is fundamentally structured on holographic principles.[7] This holds a profound implication for humanity. Not only are we physically made from the dust of stars, but our consciousness also mirrors that of the universe itself.

Once the clamour of the human ego is quietened, as happens in meditation, contemplation and prayer, we become aware of the innate spiritual quality of this consciousness – one of peace, acceptance, gratitude and love. These qualities may be felt in a bodily way. Often a person will place a hand on the heart when speaking of the soul. It is the essence of who we are. Yet the soul is not a possession like some kind of a metaphysical organ. Meister Eckhart reminds us that 'The body is much more in the soul than the soul in the body'.[8]

Until around 4000 years ago, the soul was expressed through humankind's connection with Nature. Mother Earth was very likely treated with more reverence than human life, which could be short and

---

5. See Radin (1997).
6. Bohm (1980: 125).
7. See Talbot (2011). Also discussed in *The Contribution of Spirit Release Therapy to Mental Health* and *Healing and the Wounded Psyche*, both this volume.
8. Kelley (2008: 199).

brutal. Animals, trees, mountains, valleys and rivers were regarded as emanations of spirit and honoured with ritual and ceremony through the seasons and cycles of life. The Jungian analyst Ann Baring, in her exceptional book *The Dream of the Cosmos: A Quest for the Soul*,[9] calls this participative culture the lunar era, the moon being archetypally female and a symbol of fertility.

We might be tempted to write off the lunar era as an age of superstition characterised by animistic thinking and magical propitiation of the gods. Yet it speaks of a time when 'God' had not been personified and enthroned in some far-off heaven but was manifest everywhere, and when humankind did not stand apart from the natural world but flowed with it. Several millennia later, Jesus was to point out the same when he remarked, 'Cleave the wood and I am there; lift up a stone and you will find Me there'.[10]

It is ironic that Jesus' teaching should be so at variance with the cultural epoch of his own time, for by then humankind had set its sights on taking dominion (purportedly by divine edict) 'over the fish in the sea and the birds in the sky, over the livestock and all the wild animals, and over all the creatures that move along the ground'.[11]

Baring calls this new age the solar era, in which a radical shift brought the masculine ego into the ascendant. The male principle is very dangerous when uncontained by the feminine. We have had an appalling chapter in recent history; during the 20th century, more people were killed in wars than in all of the previous known history of humankind.

The God of the Abrahamic faiths belongs to the solar era. Since it was considered that 'He' stood aside from the physical world once creation was over, there remained nothing inherently sacred about Nature. Moreover, the new image of God served as a ready projection for the exercise of institutional power and control. Women, seen as guilty by association with the temptress Eve, were excluded from clerical life and deprived of political, education and human rights, as happens in many countries to this day. Yet men have suffered too, distrust of women precluding much needed emotional intimacy and leading to sexuality being repressed or channelled into perverse outlets.

According to Christian scripture, every human being now carried the burden of sin and only baptism and divine grace could bring salvation. Little wonder, then, that when the strictures of the Church were

---

9. Baring (2013).
10. Meyer & Bloom (1993).
11. Genesis 1:26. *The Holy Bible*, NIV.

overcome in the 17th century, an Age of Enlightenment was deemed to have arrived. Notably, as the natural world opened to scientific enquiry, spirituality became disenfranchised from both Nature and daily life, with far-reaching consequences.

The stamp of material realism is now embedded deep in the culture of modernity. Material realism opened a window to a new understanding of the universe and, tragically, closed the window on the human soul.

The Age of Material Realism

The economic advantages enjoyed by high-income countries today owe more to a history of territorial conquest and economic exploitation than compassion for humankind. The great institutions of the government, the judiciary and the military ensure that social cohesion is strengthened by pulling together in the face of a common enemy, whether real or imagined. Eight trillion US dollars was spent during the Cold War and today, around 1.8 trillion dollars is being spent on arms every year.[12]

The mind of *Homo sapiens* is still evolving and has a long way to go. The problem is that the cultivation of the ego, coupled with the scientific revolution, has led to manipulation of the material world in ways hitherto unimaginable, some of which are extremely dangerous.

How can this have happened? From a neuroscience perspective, Iain McGilchrist argues in his remarkable book, *The Master and His Emissary: The Divided Brain and the Making of the Western World*, that what we are seeing is the result of a breakdown of communication between the left and right hemispheres of the brain.[13] The right cerebral hemisphere is largely concerned with the kind of consciousness that developed in the course of the lunar era as described by Baring, characterised by awareness, appreciation and integration of the whole. The left hemisphere is today the seat of ego function, language skills, problem solving and scientific analysis, all characteristic of the solar era. Unfortunately, in the course of its evolution, the left brain appears to have run away with itself and does not listen much to the right brain anymore.

Technology concerns the practical application of science to human society and is the crowning glory of the left brain. Beginning with the invention of stone tools by *Homo habilis* in the Palaeolithic era,

---

12. Shah (2013).
13. McGilchrist (2009).

technology has very likely been a powerful epigenetic spur to the advancement of human consciousness. At the same time, *Homo sapiens*, being a juvenile species in terms of planetary time and deeply impressionable, has become intoxicated with the inventions of science. Yet we cannot blame technology for even the worst crimes against humanity for, as the saying goes, a knife can be used to kill or cut bread. The problem is this: if we are to survive as a species, science needs to be taken out of the hands of the ego and put to use in the service of the soul. Otherwise, it is about as safe as giving a child a gun that fires real bullets.[14]

The Rise of Techno-pathology

I must preface this next section by emphasising that I am well aware of the countless benefits science has brought humanity. Aside from my regard for the medical sciences in general, state-of-the-art surgery some years back gave me a new lease of life for which I am profoundly grateful. However, my concern here is with the misuse of science and the extreme harm we are doing to humankind, as well as to our precious planet. I will start with a reminder of how the advance of science has influenced one lifetime – my own.

I belong to a generation that barely watched television before their teens. In my childhood, families took time to sit down to eat together, or gathered around the wireless as it was then called, with tea unhurriedly brewed in the teapot. There were two stations, the Light programme and the Home service. The broadcasts were all very innocent – no violence, just music, news, comedy and even then, the daily BBC serial *The Archers*. We children took ourselves off to the local park and strangers were not feared. Favourite toys were a Hornby clockwork train and dinky cars. There was no Top of the Pops, only a rack of much cherished gramophone records. Books were in abundance and local libraries flourished.

Nostalgia plays its part in these memories, yet I am describing a world centred on people being together and doing things together. Since there were no motorways, cars motored at a leisurely pace and

---

14. Cosmologist Stephen Hawking and Silicon Valley philanthropist Yuri Milner launched in 2016 a 100 million dollar star voyage project to pave the way for colonising the planet Proxima Centauri B, 4.2 light years from Earth (Radford, 2016). Hawking explained that there is urgency because within 100 years Earth will probably be uninhabitable. Instead of finding answers to the problems being experienced by humankind on Earth, scientists are about to export those same problems (of human nature) to another planet elsewhere in the universe.

if a person belonged to the Automobile Association, the patrol officer by the roadside would spot the badge on the car and salutes were exchanged! At the end of a train journey, we children would crowd around the big steam engine while the driver, leaning out of his cab window, would spare us a few kindly words.

Compare this with life today. One survey from the USA showed that children spend three and a half *meaningful* minutes a week talking with their parents and an average of four hours a night watching television. By the age of 11, a child will, on average, have witnessed 8000 murders on television and by 18, have watched around 200,000 violent acts on television. Two-thirds of families eat while watching television and by the age of 65, a person will have spent on average 9 years in front of the screen.[15]

Television leaves children with sensory overload together with reduced attention span.[16] Once obesity has set in, owing to physical inertia and compounded by junk food, there is even less interest in exploring into the real world. As the child's creative imagination falls into disuse, the restless mind goes channel-hopping in search of more excitement. Can we really say all this has nothing to do with the prevalence of attention deficit hyperactivity disorder (ADHD) presently recorded in children? According to the Office for National Statistics, prescriptions for the popular ADHD drug Ritalin in the UK have increased from 325,000 in 2011 to nearly 1 million in 2015.[17]

Most worrying is the relentless exposure to violence and crude sexuality. A number of studies demonstrate a clear link between early exposure to violence on screen and subsequent behaviour change, with loss of the capacity for empathy.[18] We are being shown our future, for as the poet Wordsworth observed, 'the child is father of the man',[19] not only psychologically but also in the formation of neuronal networks in the brain.

The internet has radically changed how people communicate. Letter writing has all but disappeared, and even emails are on the decline. Texting, tweeting, blogging, Skype and Facebook are the younger generation's preferred media. Many users of Facebook worry if they have fewer than 100 'friends'. How genuine are these friendships, existing

---

15. Herr (2007).
16. Contemporary programme editing ensures maximum stimulation by a technique known as 'compressed time', achieved by rapid cutting between scenes, each lasting on average seven seconds.
17. Health and Social Care Information Centre (2015: 140).
18. Anderson et al. (2010).
19. From *My Heart Leaps Up* (1802). See Wordsworth ([1994]: 91).

in a virtual domain that has no reality checks and that is based only on what people choose to post about themselves for public consumption?

There is now great concern about how the internet enables paedophiles to groom young people via 'chat rooms', apart from which there is widespread exposure to the brutalising effect of pornography. This has led to an ongoing ethical debate about the need for censorship and control, very much in contrast to the libertarian optimism of the early days of the World Wide Web.[20]

The technology of video gaming deserves special mention. It was predicted that by 2017, the global industry would reach annual sales of 109 billion US dollars.[21] It has been argued that gaming improves coordination and concentration, and that multiplayer games using sophisticated platforms enhance interactional skills. Yet more than half of the top twenty-five games being played today are dedicated to shooting and killing, while addiction to video games, known as 'problem gaming', affects up to 4% of players. Since more than 90% of young people under the age of 18 are playing video games regularly, this tells us that problem gaming must affect at least 120,000 children in the UK. One study from the USA finds that the average young person has spent 10,000 hours of gaming by the age of 21,[22] the same length of time it takes to become a concert pianist or a world-class athlete.

In 2012, the UK charity Childline received 1.5 million contacts from children in distress.[23] The main reasons for seeking help were:

- family relationship problems (up 18% on the year before), notably with communication problems cited most often: 195,000 contacts
- physical and sexual abuse: 165,000 contacts
- bullying (including cyber-bullying and cyber-blackmail): 150,000 contacts
- self-harming (up 68%): 75,000 contacts
- depression and mental health problems (up 19%): 75,000 contacts
- risk of suicide (up 39%): 60,000 contacts.

Whatever other benefits technology may bring, it does not seem to have helped the world of the child to become a happier, more secure and nurturing environment.[24]

---

20. The increasing use of the internet to groom for terrorism purposes has only served to heighten this debate.
21. McDonald (2017).
22. A statistic celebrated by McGonigal (2011), who is a keen advocate of gaming.
23. For the year 2014/2015, the Childline website received 3.2 million visits and counselling was provided for 300,000 children. See NSPCC (2015).
24. A longitudinal follow-up study of 19,000 children born in 2000–2001, reports

The consumer society is the shop window of secular technology. Consumerism promises happiness but the best it can give is pleasure, and when the excitement of the latest 'must-have' is over, the need for the next one takes its place. Compulsive pleasure-seeking has the same root cause as much alcohol and substance misuse, which is to ward off feelings of emptiness and futility. As such, it can never compensate for the pleasure in helping others, the valuing of kinship, the lightness of heart that comes with honesty and openness, the appreciation of the gift of life and joy in the beauty of the natural world. These spiritual attributes are of the soul, awakened by loving relationships for which no machine or electronic device can substitute. The less time that is found for face-to-face human intimacy, the more impoverished the child and the greater the handicap for the adult in the making.

Without going further into developmental psychology, it is easy to see how growing up in a world of things rather than people[25] can leave a person unskilled at relating, unconfident of love and vulnerable to depression, eating disorders and substance misuse. There is now an epidemic of mental health disorders in the UK.[26] One in five people will be diagnosed with depression during their lifetime, with rates for women twice those for men.[27] Overall, there are more than 5500 suicides per year in this country.[28] Eating disorders currently run at 750,000 for the UK.[29] 9% of adult men and 4% of adult women show alcohol dependence, with over 21,000 people dying each year due to alcohol-related events,[30] while around 10% of the population of the UK take illicit drugs resulting in over 2500 deaths per year.[31]

In some areas, the benefits of scientific enterprise appear to be unarguable, for instance, the provision of clean running water, sanitation, the technology of food production and life-saving advances in

---

that 1 in 4 girls and 1 in 10 boys aged 14 years are depressed. See UCL Centre for Longitudinal Studies (2017).

25. The theologian Martin Buber uses two word-pairs to describe human life. The 'I-It' describes how we experience an object (thing) that is separate in itself. This is the foundation of science. The 'I-Thou' describes an attitude that does not objectify but acknowledges and finds meaning in all living relationships and ultimately (for Buber) in relation to God. See Buber (2013).
26. For a full update, see Mental Health Foundation (2016). Also detailed in *Recovery and Well-Being: The Search for the Soul*, this volume.
27. Health and Social Care Information Centre (2014).
28. According to the Office for National Statistics (2016), 5688 suicides were recorded in 2016 in the UK for people aged 15 and older; of these, some 75% were male and 25% were female.
29. BEAT survey (BEAT, 2015).
30. Alcohol Concern (2016).
31. Office for National Statistics (2015).

medical care. At the same time, we need to think hard about the consequences of even these most benign technologies.

The Population Explosion

By removing the checks and balances that Nature applied to the human species over hundreds of thousands of years, advances first in agriculture, then in industry and now in healthcare have triggered a steep rise in the human population. Our species has grown from 1 million 10,000 years ago, to 1 billion 200 years ago, to over 7 billion today. Just supporting this number, let alone future growth, is destroying the Earth's ecology. Stephen Emmott[32] offers a daunting analysis of the current degradation of the planet's ecosystem – the atmosphere, hydrosphere (the planet's water), cryosphere (ice sheets and glaciers) and biosphere (plants and animals). Some of the evidence Emmott provides has been challenged, but the fact remains that eco-scientists are deeply worried.

We now have toxic levels of the greenhouse gases, carbon dioxide, methane and nitrous oxide. Global temperatures are rising, accompanied by extreme weather conditions, with severe floods and droughts. The oceans are warming, fish stocks have been decimated and biodiversity is plummeting, with accelerating species' extinction. Tropical forest and woodland is shrinking and global fresh water supplies are failing. Despite this, more cars, ships and planes are being made than ever before and energy demands continue to soar.[33] In the UK, the government has approved nationwide fracking for natural gas.

People respond in different ways, from outright denial to deep concern. Some are prepared to take any measures that may help, including civil disobedience. Some are happy to sign up to the 'green' economy but do not go much beyond that. Others are resigned to the view that nothing can stop the inevitable and that all we can do is live on borrowed time. Not least, there are opportunists behind the scenes who continue to manipulate the system for power and profit. Speaking up about this can make a person sound like the victim of conspiracy

---

32. Emmott (2013).
33. The greenhouse gas emissions of the meat industry are greater than those produced by the sum of all plane, train, car, lorry and boat transportations. While methane produced by livestock agriculture amounts to only around 18% of global greenhouse gas emissions (compared with fossil fuel and industrial processes, which generate over two-thirds), methane traps up to 100 times more heat in the atmosphere than carbon dioxide within a five-year period. See US Environmental Protection Agency (2014).

theory. Nevertheless, such machinations of self-interest and unconcern for the fate of humanity represent the egotistical extreme of the solar era, despite the endeavours of other good-hearted people doing their best for humanity.

The Breakdown of Trust

Peter Joseph, who directed the controversial documentary-style *Zeitgeist: The Movie*,[34] was roundly condemned for his critique of the history of duplicity and corruption in the Catholic Church; the claim that the US government was forewarned of the attacks on 9/11 but did nothing, so that there could be justification for a subsequent War on Terror; and that a cabal of international bankers effectively rule the world by manipulating money markets with complete indifference to human suffering. Blending fact and fiction is a dangerous gambit, but in excess of 50 million people have viewed *Zeitgeist* and this 'docufiction' has only served to deepen distrust of the great political, economic, military and religious institutions. There has since been the revelation of child sex abuse in the Catholic Church, the world has suffered a global banking crisis and the War on Terror, which looks to be of indefinite duration, funds ever more advanced weapons technology.[35]

Disinformation is commonplace in the corridors of power. One tactic is to dismiss investigative reporting as paranoid scaremongering. The secrecy surrounding geoengineering projects, as highlighted by GeoEngineering Watch,[36] illustrates the problem. Take, for instance, the construction of High Frequency Active Auroral Research Program (HAARP) in Alaska. An array of 180 radio antennas spread over 33 acres is capable of beaming a signal of 3.6 million watts modulated to extremely low frequency (ELF) into the ionosphere. This instrument allegedly has the power to punch holes in clouds, divert hurricanes, create storms, trigger earthquakes and tsunamis, and target and destroy communications systems anywhere in the world. The consortium that funded this project and in which the US military have the largest share, is unaccountable to the wider electorate. HAARP is acknowledged to exist, its stated purpose being to develop ionospheric enhancement

---

34. Joseph (2007).
35. World military expenditure is estimated to have been 1676 billion US dollars in 2015, amounting to 2.3% of global gross domestic product or 228 dollars per person. See *SIPRI Yearbook* (Stockholm International Peace Research Institute, 2016: 17).
36. GeoEngineering Watch (2017).

technology for radio communications and surveillance. Charges that it has been used as a military weapon or for solar radiation management are strongly denied.

A second example of geoengineering concerns alleged 'chemtrails'. These are described as similar to the condensation trails created by jet aircraft but, unlike ordinary vapour trails that disperse, a chemtrail is formed by releasing an aerosol containing nanoparticles of heavy metals such as aluminium and barium that persist in the upper atmosphere. The sky becomes a patchwork quilt of trails, which gradually merge into cirrus-like clouds that can last for days. The aim is said to be to reduce global warming, the cloud layer of aluminium particles reducing the penetration of sunlight. Chemtrails are conceded as a potential strategy for solar radiation management by the geoengineering lobby, although there is blanket denial that they are already in use. Nevertheless, dozens of videos of alleged chemtrails filmed by eco-activists can be seen on YouTube. There are numerous reports of dying trees and vegetation in North America and Canada, and rainfall tested in Australia has showed high levels of neurotoxic heavy metals, including aluminium, manganese and boron. Manganese is an electrical conductant that enhances the carriage of extra-low frequency radio waves and it is claimed that it is being added to chemtrails to potentiate transmissions from HAARP. Boron induces male sterility at high doses and this has raised fears that it is being covertly tested in population-control programmes.

These are extreme views that most people would find incredible. Nevertheless, concerning aluminium, it is a fact that in 2009, a US gene patent for aluminium-resistant seeds was granted.[37] Worryingly, nanoparticles of aluminium readily cross the blood-brain barrier and we know that aluminium is implicated in neurological degenerative disorders including Alzheimer's disease,[38] which now affects one person in three over the age of 80.

Not surprisingly, such alarms are dismissed by sceptics as scaremongering typical of conspiracy theorists. On the other side, activists are convinced they have lifted the lid on nefarious operations being carried out by a covert elite unaccountable to public office. Extreme claims have been made, for instance, that the USA used HAARP to trigger the Japan earthquake of 11 March 2011.[39] What motive could

---

37. For the technically minded, see US Patent Office (2007). For the non-technical, see GeoEngineering Watch (2014).
38. Kawahara & Kato-Negishi (2011).
39. Magnetometer readings from HAARP showed broadcasting at 2.5 kHz, a known seismic-inducing wavelength, from 8 to 11 March precisely. Just prior to the earthquake, luminescent cloud formations typical of those generated

there possibly be? It has been alleged that the USA was determined to stop an imminent trade agreement between Iran and Japan that would trade nuclear technology for oil (Japan is dependent on Iran for oil, taking 12% of Iran's annual production).

What are we to believe? Human beings are capable of doing very good things and very bad things and we have to decide on the evidence for ourselves. Either way, there is now a major problem of lack of trust. If a person does challenge the status quo, he or she will be seen as paranoid, gullible or plain eccentric. All this may be true, but it does not necessarily mean the person is wrong. It is a sobering thought that one person in twenty-five is a sociopath[40] and that clever, ambitious sociopaths relish nothing more than wielding power.

Finally, there is the problem of nuclear technology. Aside from the insane current stockpile of 17,000 warheads (94% of which are American or Russian) and the risk from terrorism or computer malfunction, we are now living with the consequences of the meltdowns at the Chernobyl and Fukushima nuclear power plants.

The Soviet Union did not report the Chernobyl disaster of 1986 (it was left to Sweden), and people living in the area were not given potassium iodide tablets to protect them against the cloud of radioactive iodine-131. Over 6000 have developed thyroid cancer to date.[41] One study, carried out by Alexey Yablokov, President of the Russian Centre for Environmental Policy, predicts an eventual excess mortality close to 1 million worldwide due to the global radioactive fallout.[42] The Chernobyl reactor core was eventually sealed inside a massive concrete sarcophagus. However, within a few years this began to degrade because of water penetration.[43]

The Fukushima Daiichi disaster in Japan in 2011 has left 10 million people living in highly radioactive areas, and around 37,000 children have already been found on scanning to have developed thyroid

---

      by HAARP were seen over Japan, accompanied by a sudden rise in the electron content of the ionosphere over its epicentre. For an example of a post-Fukushima activist blog, see Socio-Economics History Blog (2011), and for a 'conspiracy theory' compilation, see YouTube (2012).

40.   Stout (2006).
41.   Lisbeth Gronlund, senior scientist and co-director of the Union of Concerned Scientists (UCS), calculates that in addition to thyroid cancer, between 27,000 and 53,000 excess cancers and cancer deaths will be attributable to Chernobyl. By 2005, some 6000 thyroid cancers had already been diagnosed. Gronlund (2011).
42.   Yablokov et al. (2010).
43.   A new sarcophagus, costing 1.5 billion dollars, was completed in 2017, intended to last 100 years.

nodules.[44] The meltdown at Fukushima was three times worse than Chernobyl and radioactive waste is still pouring into the sea. There remains the likelihood of further meltdown if there is another explosive release of hydrogen gas, or more seismic activity. There is no way to decommission either Chernobyl or Fukushima. Both will remain intensely radioactive for millennia.

Conflicting World-views

Most of us are too busy getting on with daily life to think much about things like geoengineering and nuclear fallout. That was true for me until I began to do some research for a paper I was giving. Looking into the 'dark side' of technology, I found myself caught between two opposing realities – that of the so-called conspiracy theorists, and that of the sceptics who claimed to represent normality. The existential impact was even more disturbing since, as shown in the Gestalt image of 'old woman/young woman', it proved impossible to hold both perspectives without the one negating the other.

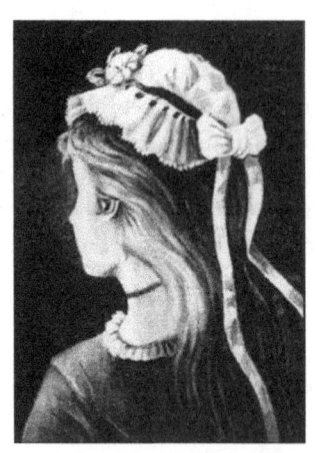

14.1 Gestalt figure/ground reversal
(anonymous German postcard, c. 1888).

Because it is so difficult to get a hold on reality when it comes to disinformation and conspiracy theory, it is not surprising that the climate is one of suspicion, even paranoia. I am reminded of having once asked a sheep farmer why his sheep grazed happily in the field without straying through holes in the hedge. He explained, 'One in a hundred sheep, usually a tup (the ram), finds the holes. Then the others all follow'. I asked him what he did about it. He replied, 'We take out the tup!'

---

44. For a comprehensive medical update, see Rosen & Claussen (2016).

In this situation, psychological defences come into play. A person may be in denial, either because it is too scary to contemplate the sinister scenario, or more generally, because it challenges the consensus reality on which a person's customary identity depends. Consequently, trying to fathom what is really happening can be hard. Is the so-called 'conspiracy theorist' like the tup who finds the hole in the hedge or is this nothing more than alarmism, leading people mistakenly to see elephants in an empty room?

There is no question that a dark side to technology exists. We know how the internet is used for fraud, paedophilia and, increasingly, terrorism. Scientists of public renown like Michio Kaku are warning us of this.[45] Just how close are we to George Orwell's 'big brother' future world dystopia?[46] Each of us has to make their own determination, but at the least, we should be willing to take a good look through the hole in the hedge!

Engaging the Soul

If we try to oppose techno-pathology, we face a particular challenge. Any activism in which the egoic self is invested will always run into opposition (as the saying goes, one man's terrorist is another man's freedom fighter). This is in accordance with Newton's third law of motion, which states that for every action, there is an equal and opposite reaction.[47]

The ego likes nothing better than a good fight in a good cause. Yet by engaging in mental combat, even with the best of intentions, we end up battling with dualities from which there is no escape. The control and command dynamics of the solar era will always ensure that dissenters like Bradley Manning[48] and Edward Snowden[49] are vilified and prosecuted without mercy.

---

45. *The Dark Side of Technology* by Michio Kaku (2012).
46. Orwell (1949).
47. No matter how near we may stand to the light, the ego cannot help but cast its shadow. However, the soul, being itself of the light, is beyond duality, as are its emanations.
48. Military whistle-blower Bradley Manning (now Chelsea Manning) was given a 35-year prison sentence after being convicted of leaking classified military material to Julian Assange's site WikiLeaks in 2013. She was released in 2017, following commutation of the sentence by President Obama.
49. Edward Snowden, former US Intelligence Community Officer, leaked documents in 2013 opening a public window into the National Security Agency's international intelligence partners' secret mass surveillance programmes and capabilities. He has been granted asylum in Russia.

It is clear to me that science and technology are fuelling a runaway train in which the driver has become intoxicated with power and speed. The passengers travelling first class are enjoying good food and fine wine, and the view from the observation car. The economy class cannot afford to eat, but human companionship (and sex) does not cost anything. Some passengers have realised the train is out of control and are praying to God to step in and apply the brakes. Others are beseeching the driver to slow down but he can't or won't listen – such is the inflation of the ego.

If arm-twisting makes no impression, nor the ringing of alarm bells, premonitions of doom and even the fear of death, what else may be done? As all who value the spiritual life[50] know, there is another way, but it requires humanity to listen to the soul. Where the ego seeks to be loved, the soul's desire is to love. The volatile emotions of the mundane life hold no attraction for the soul, which quietly continues to find expression in joyfulness, gratitude, compassion and kindness. None of these qualities can be weighed or measured, and they are therefore destined to remain beyond the reach of empirical science. Yet the non-personal, non-conditional benevolence of spiritual love can touch the hardest of hearts.

Since the vision of the soul is unitive, there is no question of wrestling the ego out of the way. Neither does the soul measure its actions by calculation of success or failure; it continues in the only way it knows how, which is to disarm with kindness and compassion.

Fortunately, since the ego seeks love, it is susceptible to the influence of the soul and while it may be a slow learner, it is not ineducable. Herein lies the future of humanity – if there is to be one.

As far as saving the planet goes, there are countless activists working on carbon emissions, renewable resources and the like, all of which is good and necessary. Nevertheless, I am suggesting that how we go about it is of the essence. I have cautioned that when action is ego-driven, opposition is inevitable. However, when action is soul-inspired, there is no battle to win, only loving concern for the good of all. Then the way is open to finding understanding, overcoming divisions and reconciling opposites, trusting that in its own time and in its own way, the outcome will be good.[51]

According to folklore, we are all flowers in God's garden – one very big garden, infinitely large in fact. If we can learn to harness the

---

50. This does not entail rejecting the material world; the spiritual life is simply one in which spiritual reality means more to a person than material reality.
51. Cf. the parable of the sower: 'Still other seed fell on good soil. It came up, grew and produced a crop, some multiplying thirty, some sixty, some a hundred times'. Mark 4:8. *The Holy Bible*, NIV.

achievements of science with the soul values of inclusiveness, harmony, wholeness and love, in this decisive age for humanity we will have helped tend a garden that may yet flourish.

The evolution of social history is mirrored in the maturation of the individual. The world of the child is lunar in its sense of timelessness, mystery and wonder. Then, with progressive mastery of the environment, the ego embarks on a journey into the solar world. Later in life, the pace eases and the lunar returns, a precious opportunity to become more cognisant of the soul's wisdom.

May humanity avail itself of this wisdom while it can! Left to the devices of the ego, humankind will destroy itself with the technology we have at our disposal today. In the time that remains, let us pray that we shall learn how to use technology in the service of the soul.

References

Alcohol Concern (2016) Alcohol statistics. Available at: https://www.alcoholconcern.org.uk/alcohol-statistics (accessed 8 July 2107).

Anderson, C.A., Shibuya. A., Ihori, N., et al. (2010) Violent video game effects on aggression, empathy, and prosocial behavior in Eastern and Western countries: a meta-analytic review. *Psychological Bulletin*, 136, 151–173.

Baring, A. (2013) *The Dream of the Cosmos: A Quest for the Soul.* Archive Publishing.

BEAT (2015) Statistics for journalists. BEAT. Available at: https://www.b-eat.co.uk/about-beat/media-centre/information-and-statistics-about-eating-disorders (accessed 8 July 2017).

Bohm, D. (1980) *Wholeness and the Implicate Order.* Routledge.

Buber, M. (2013) *I and Thou.* Bloomsbury Academic.

Emmott, S. (2013) *10 Billion.* Penguin Books.

Gardner, F. (2016) *The Only Mind Worth Having: Thomas Merton and the Child's Mind.* Lutterworth Press.

GeoEngineering Watch (2014) Chemtrails killing organic crops, Monsanto's GMO seeds thrive. GeoEngineering Watch, 23 May. Available at http://www.geoengineeringwatch.org/chemtrails-killing-organic-crops-monsantos-gmo-seeds-thrive/ (accessed 8 July 2017).

GeoEngineering Watch (2017) Want to know about HAARP? GeoEngineering Watch. Available at: http://www.geoengineeringwatch.org/want-to-know-about-haarp/ (accessed 8 July 2017).

Gronlund, L. (2011) How many cancers did Chernobyl really cause? (updated version). Union of Concerned Scientists. Available at: http://allthingsnuclear.org/lgronlund/how-many-cancers-did-chernobyl-really-cause-updated (accessed 8 July 2017).

Health and Social Care Information Centre (2014) *Health Survey for England.* HSCIC. Available at: http://healthsurvey.hscic.gov.uk/support-guidance/public-health/health-survey-for-england-2014/mental-health-problems.aspx (accessed 8 July 2017).

Health and Social Care Information Centre (2015) *Prescriptions Dispensed in the Community, Statistics for England – 2004–2014*. HSCIC. Available at: http://content.digital.nhs.uk/catalogue/PUB17644/pres-disp-com-eng-2004-14-rep.pdf (accessed 8 July 2017).

Herr, N. (2007) Television & health. California State University. Available at: https://www.csun.edu/science/health/docs/tv&health.html#tv_stats (accessed 8 July 2017).

Joseph, P. (2007) *Zeitgeist: The Movie*. Available at: https://www.youtube.com/watch?v=pTbIu8Zeqp0 (accessed 8 July 2017).

Kaku, M. (2012) *The Dark Side of Technology*. Available at: https://www.youtube.com/watch?v=dTi4v3HveqE (accessed 8 July 2017).

Kawahara, M. & Kato-Negishi, M. (2011) Link between aluminum and the pathogenesis of Alzheimer's disease: the integration of the aluminum and amyloid cascade hypotheses. *International Journal of Alzheimer's Disease*, 2, 1–17.

Kelley, C. (2008) *Meister Eckhart on Divine Knowledge*. Frog.

McDonald, E. (2017) The global games market will reach $108.9 billion in 2017 with mobile taking 42% - Newzoo, Gamesindustry.biz, 20 April. Available at: https://newzoo.com/insights/articles/the-global-games-market-will-reach-108-9-billion-in-2017-with-mobile-taking-42/ (accessed 8 July 2017).

McGilchrist, I. (2009) *The Master and His Emissary: The Divided Brain and the Making of the Western World*. Yale University Press.

McGonigal, J. (2011) *Reality is Broken: Why Games Make Us Better and How They Can Change the World*. Penguin Books.

Mental Health Foundation (2016) *Fundamental Facts about Mental Health*. Mental Health Foundation. Available at: https://www.mentalhealth.org.uk/sites/default/files/fundamental-facts-about-mental-health-2016.pdf (accessed 8 July 2017).

Meyer, M. & Bloom, H. (1993) *Gospel of Thomas* (Saying 77). Bravo.

NSPCC (2015) *'Always There When I Need You': Childline Annual Review 2014–15. What Children are Contacting Childline About*. NSPCC. Available at: https://www.nspcc.org.uk/services-and-resources/research-and-resources/2015/childline-annual-review-2014-2015-always-there/ (accessed 8 July 2017).

Office for National Statistics (2015) Deaths related to drug poisoning in England and Wales: 2015 registrations. ONS. Available at: https://www.ons.gov.uk/peoplepopulationandcommunity/birthsdeathsandmarriages/deaths/bulletins/deathsrelatedtodrugpoisoninginenglandandwales/2015registrations#main-points (accessed 8 July 2107).

Office for National Statistics (2016) Suicides in Great Britain: 2016 registrations. ONS. Available at: https://www.ons.gov.uk/peoplepopulationandcommunity/birthsdeathsandmarriages/deaths/bulletins/suicidesintheunitedkingdom/2016registration/previous/v1 (accessed 8 July 2017).

Orwell, G. (1949) *Nineteen Eighty-Four*. Penguin Classics.

Radford, T. (2016) Stephen Hawking and Yuri Milner launch $100m star voyage. *The Guardian*, 12 April. Available at: https://www.theguardian.com/science/2016/apr/12/stephen-hawking-and-yuri-milner-launch-100m-star-voyage (accessed 13 September 2017).

Radin, D. (1997) *The Conscious Universe*. HarperCollins.

Rosen, A. & Claussen, A. (2016) *5 Years Living With Fukushima: Summary of the Health Effects of the Nuclear Catastrophe*. IPPNW Germany. Available at: http://www.psr.org/assets/pdfs/fukushima-report.pdf (accessed 8 July 2017).

Samples, B. (1976) *The Metaphoric Mind: a Celebration of Creative Consciousness*. Longman Publishing.
Shah, A. (2013) World military spending. Global Issues (updated 30 June 2013). Available at: http://www.globalissues.org/article/75/world-military-spending#WorldMilitarySpending (accessed 8 July 2017).
Socio-Economics History Blog (2011) HAARP magnetometer data shows Japan earthquake was induced! socioecohistory.wordpress.com, 28 March. Available at: https://socioecohistory.wordpress.com/2011/03/28/haarp-magnetometer-data-shows-japan-earthquake-was-induced/ (accessed 13 September 2017).
Stockholm International Peace Research Institute (2016) *SIPRI Yearbook: Armaments, Disarmament and International Security*. SIPRI. Available at: https://www.sipri.org/sites/default/files/YB16-Summary-ENG.pdf (accessed 20 September 2017).
Stout, M. (2006) *The Sociopath Next Door*. Broadway Books.
Talbot, M. (2011) *The Holographic Universe: The Revolutionary Theory of Reality*. Harper Perennial.
UCL Centre for Longitudinal Studies (2017) *Millennium Study*. UCL. Available at: http://www.cls.ioe.ac.uk/ (accessed 20 September 2017).
US Environmental Protection Agency (2014) Global greenhouse gas emissions data. USEPA. Available at: https://www.epa.gov/ghgemissions/global-greenhouse-gas-emissions-data (accessed 8 July 2017).
US Patent Office (2007) Sorghum aluminum tolerance gene, SbMATE (Publication Number 7582809 B2). Available at: http://www.google.co.uk/patents/US7582809 (accessed 13 September 2017).
Wordsworth, W. (1994) *The Collected Poems of William Wordsworth*. Wordsworth Editions.
Yablokov, A., Nesterenko, V. & Nesterenko, A. (2010) *Chernobyl: Consequences of the Catastrophe for People and the Environment*. Annals of the New York Academy of Sciences. Wiley-Blackwell.
YouTube (2012) *HAARP: Japan 2011 (Proof)*. Available at: https://www.youtube.com/watch?v=R66-9hDhfpw (accessed 8 July 2017).

15

Modernity and the Beleaguered Soul

The title of this paper is intended to convey what I see as a deep prejudice in today's world towards matters of the soul. As a consequence, we are living in both a dangerous and endangered world, not because people are any worse than they used to be, but because we now have powerful technologies at our fingertips that the ego, without the benefit of the soul, does not understand how to use with discernment.

I first want to explore the impact of the scientific world-view on humankind, one that began with the European Renaissance and which now, through the outreach of technology, extends across the globe. Yet the excesses of the ego were in evidence long before the scientific revolution, and so I first need to begin with the great religions, whose spiritual aim has been all too often derailed by incursions of the human ego, thereby creating not unity but division.

I shall then highlight how the discoveries of science, which to begin with had no argument with a spiritual cosmology, developed a materialist narrative that estranged science from religion. In pursuit of this, the human ego made its mark by turning science into 'scientism' – the all-pervasive myth of our time and now the mainstay of a society geared to financial power, profit, perpetual debt and, on a deeper level, one of terrifying meaninglessness.[1]

Finally, I will explore some of the social consequences of the current multibillion dollar 'persuasion industry'. I do not only mean the rampant marketing of consumables and luxuries, but also the dominance of political, military, economic and industrial power-broking,

---

Paper prepared for the 4th British Congress on Medicine and Spirituality, London, November 2013.

---

1. Scientism: the belief that empirical science constitutes the most authoritative world-view to the extent that other perspectives are devalued or altogether excluded.

and to illustrate how pervasive mechanisms of control work today through being extensively woven into our technology.

The bad news is that since our minds have been conditioned from childhood not to question many of the assumptions that govern our behaviour, we are more captive to cultural norms than we know. The good news, however, is that the soul is impervious to the manipulations of the ego and remains a precious source of wisdom, provided we turn to it for counsel. On this more optimistic note, I shall argue that our best hope for the future lies not in looking outwards for signposts but in looking inwards, by paying attention to the soul.

The Soul in Search of a Home

Throughout history, the great spiritual masters have constantly encouraged humanity to heed the soul. The essence of their teachings centres on the virtue and value of love as expressed in kindness, compassion and care for all of life. The task may seem hopeless but, as Jesus remarked, a grain of mustard grows into a tree in which the birds of the air make their nests.[2] Spiritual teachings have been disseminated over recent millennia through a number of established religions. Broadly speaking, of the current world population of 7.5 billion, some 30% are Christian, 25% Muslim, 15% Hindu and 7% Buddhist, not counting many other faith traditions with worldwide followings, including Judaism and Spiritism, each of which numbers around 0.2%.[3]

We are indebted to the great religions for their profound moral and cultural heritage, and their fostering of the arts, literature and education. In the more recent history of the West, religion has been prominent in social reform, including the abolition of slavery and the advancement of human rights. However, the history of humanity, going back to Sumerian and Egyptian times and including the classical antiquity of Greece and Rome, is not a story of harmony among nations or peoples. Throughout the ages, religion has not delivered 'peace on earth and goodwill to all men' and given the conflict-ridden state of the world today, it is hard to imagine how it can ever do so.

Acts of human intolerance and aggression carried out in the name of religion have, of course, nothing to do with the original spiritual teachings. In such cases, religion has been hijacked to serve other interests,

---

2. Luke 13:18–21. *The Holy Bible*, NIV.
3. Pew Research Center (2017).

something that happens all the more readily if a given religion regards itself as possessing a truth greater than others.[4] The ego latches on to this; hence the shocking history of converting unbelievers by force, of which a number of religions are guilty.

Such religious splits and factions have resulted in a trail of destruction. Christians invaded Muslim territories in the Crusades; throughout the Inquisition the Catholic Church tortured thousands of so-called heretics; Catholics and Protestants fought it out in Northern Ireland; now Shia and Sunni Muslims are doing the same in Syria and elsewhere, while in India, Muslims and Hindus continue to murder each other.[5]

Nevertheless, rather than condemn religion, as self-proclaimed atheist and author Richard Dawkins does in *The God Delusion*,[6] we can appreciate that religious beliefs arise from a deep yearning within the human spirit. From the dawn of history, certainly since Neolithic times, there has been a spiritual impulse that impels humankind to seek a greater reality, one that transcends the whys and wherefores of everyday life. But for this, the great religions could never have flourished.

Yet there are problems, for in the acquisition of institutional powers, religious orthodoxy can become more sacrosanct than personal revelation. Indeed, many clerics are nervous of epiphanies that might turn out to be subversive, which is why prophets, seers and sages have generally had a hard time of it.

Most people are not visionaries and are happy enough to follow the guidance of their religious leaders. More recently, however, the UK National Census revealed a marked decline in religious observance. Although 60% of British still describe themselves as Christian, the majority are over 60 years of age, and church membership has declined from 30% of the population in 1930 to 10% in 2013, with regular church attendance down to 5%.[7] Does this mean the general population is less spiritual than previously? I do not think so, as I shall be discussing shortly.

---

4. The possible exception is Buddhism (although not everyone sees Buddhism as a religion). The Buddha advised people to try Buddhism and see if it worked for them – if not, to try something else!
5. Sectarian terrorism is now world-wide. The global *jihad* mounted by the self-proclaimed Islamic State of Iraq and the Levant (ISIL) has led to a crisis unparalleled in history. For a concise summary, see report by Council on Foreign Relations (Laub, 2016).
6. Dawkins (2007).
7. *Faith Survey* including statistics from the UK National Census of 2011. See Brierley Consultancy (2016).

Mechanistic Science and the Rise of Secularism

Before the scientific revolution, religion shaped the aspirations of humankind. The worldly hierarchy of power and authority was mirrored in the hierarchy of the heavenly host, commanded by God. People generally believed there was a rightful order of things, which included being born into their station in life and mostly staying there. Theological assertions were absolute and not to be questioned, including the geocentric movements of the heavenly bodies.

With the advent of science all this changed. Although the origins of modernity can be found in the work of Copernicus, Kepler and Galileo, the revolutionary world-view dates from the publication of Isaac Newton's *Principia* in 1687, describing a universe in which mathematical principles accounted for the motion of planets. Newton was deeply religious and saw no contradiction between his laws of physics and a creator God. He wrote that '...the motions which the planets now have could not spring from any natural cause alone, but were impressed by an intelligent Agent... not blind and fortuitous, but very well skilled in Mechanicks and Geometry'.[8] However, the impact of Newton's scientific method inspired a new breed of natural scientists who dared suppose that one day the human intellect would be able to explain everything about the universe.

As the scientific exploration of Nature gathered pace, the eclectic pursuits of Renaissance man were succeeded by the emerging disciplines of mathematics, physics, chemistry, botany and zoology, each in turn differentiating into the vast array of specialisations we have today. There is no aspect of the material world, animal, vegetable or mineral, that has been overlooked, from the outer reaches of the galaxy to the arcane mysteries of particle physics. Except for pure mathematics and psychology, which deal in abstractions, science addresses physical reality. Yet the unforeseen consequence of the scientific method has been such that in just a few hundred years, humankind has set itself apart from the flow and rhythm of the natural world, which is now seen as being there principally to serve the needs of the human species.

Step by step, we humans of the modern age have had our worldview shaped by science so that we no longer question its assumptions about the nature of reality. Science assumes that events take place by chance, unless they are found to be clustered together in such a way as to be amenable to experimental replication, in which case they are considered 'meaningful'. This is the basis of statistics. From an ocean

---

8. Heller (2009: 148).

of apparently random events, natural laws can then be identified and used to test theories. The whole idea is to demonstrate and explain how things happen. The experimenter, who must be separate from the thing being observed, sets about compiling a data set. If an experiment is repeated ten times with the same result, it is noteworthy. If it can be repeated 100 times, people start talking about something having been proved. It is a numbers game that does not set much store by what an individual experiences.

Classical physics holds that there is a fixed, immutable 'reality' out there, and that each of us passes through it on the timeline of birth to death. Everything has a timeline, even our universe, which began 13.7 billion years ago and will end in what is called 'heat death' in 10^{150} years. Our little solar system makes a brief appearance, being just over 4.5 billion years old and already in its midlife. In about 1 billion years from now, the oceans of Earth will evaporate as the sun turns into a red giant, eventually engulfing all its planets before cooling to the point of extinction.

For good reason, mechanistic science has progressively dominated the world-view of human beings over the past three centuries. First, it explains a great deal about the physical world. Second, it creates a sense of security; no longer is humankind in thrall to the mysterious workings of a supreme deity.[9] Third, science has spawned a massive technology on which we depend, from steam to electricity, from the silicon chip to the Large Hadron Collider. Along with a mass of appliances that populate our homes, there are machines that transport us by land, sea and air, keep us alive in hospital, plough fields and plant crops – the list is endless.

Yet if life is merely a biological event taking place in a mechanistic universe, there are some profound implications. Birth is down to chance; death is final; consciousness is simply a by-product of brain activity; there is no actual purpose in life; suffering is meaningless and love is nothing more than Nature's way of ensuring pair bonding and the procreation of the species.

There are social consequences, too. Go pleasure seeking (you may as well have a good time while it lasts); work for material success (it gets you status, makes you money and can buy you pleasure); if you feel empty or at a loss, alcohol or drugs are on hand to ward off unwelcome thoughts and feelings (such as asking yourself what it is all for); have as

---

9. Instead, we have the new religion of scientism, inculcated from a young age and thereafter rarely questioned. For a penetrating cultural analysis, see Sheldrake (2012).

much sex as you can (it is a good short-acting antidepressant); expose yourself to violence on-screen (it excites the animal instincts and makes you feel more alive – or at least less deadened).[10]

Science is supposed to be free from value judgements and to be concerned only with finding out how things work. Yet humanity has gorged itself unthinkingly on the fruits of science and technology.[11] The ego has gone on a shopping spree in search of new gods – from designer clothes to trading in one's smartphone for an upgrade with more apps you don't need, or buying a car that goes faster than you will ever drive, usually with money you don't have. Never mind about that, just borrow today and pay back some other time![12]

Consider what it means these days to buy a home on a mortgage. A person can proudly say, 'This is *my* home'. In fact, the home really belongs to the bank that has just lent you a large sum of money. The bank will go on to make a lot more money out of you for having done nothing except lend you money in the first place – virtual money, incidentally, that the bank does not actually possess – and will then take your home away if you do not, or cannot, pay up.

The world of material realism has created untold opportunities for making money out of others. This would be no different from the pyramid selling scandals that used to do the rounds years ago, except for the excuse that in a growth economy *everyone* is supposed to get rich. This has worked for only so long as Earth could be treated as an unlimited resource, like a bank with infinite money supply. Now we know different. As Mahatma Gandhi is said to have remarked, the world has enough for everyone's need, but never enough for everyone's greed.

We cannot blame science any more than we should blame religion for the mess we are in today. Responsibility for the state of the world must lie with the human species, driven by the short-sighted ambitions of the human ego. Technology has enslaved rather than liberated, blunted rather than enhanced consciousness. Only now as we become aware of the full impact of what we have been doing do we begin to see that we have put at risk our own survival.

---

10. Worse still, exposure to violence has been shown to impair the capacity for empathy. Guo et al. (2013).
11. See *Technology and Soul in the 21ˢᵗ Century*, this volume.
12. Personal debt in the UK now runs at 1.43 trillion pounds sterling. Report by the Centre for Social Justice (2013).

Science and Spirituality Today

From the mechanistic perspective, the second law of thermodynamics tells us that, like a clock winding down, everything eventually must stop. Nevertheless, questions remain. How did the clock wind itself up in the first place? What was there before it started ticking? What happens after it stops? This is where Newtonian physics gets stuck, because its concept of reality is confined to measurement of the physical universe.

To go beyond these horizons requires entirely new ways of thinking. For example, Professor Wun-Yi Shu has put forward a cosmological theory in which the speed of light and the gravitational constant are both variable and time has no beginning or end. At a certain point, time converts into space, while mass converts into length, and the universe begins to expand. At another point, the opposite goes on: length converts to mass and space into time, and the universe contracts.[13] There is no cosmic arrow of time, no beginning and no end, but instead, an oscillation of expansion and contraction in perpetuity, much as in Hindu mythology – the universe giving birth to form with each outbreath and reclaiming it with each inbreath.

Shu's theory as yet fails to account for the background cosmic microwave radiation that is thought to be left over from the Big Bang. However, if Shu is right, both Einstein's gravitational constant and the fixed speed of light would turn out to be transient phenomena in the greater scheme of things.

Stephen Hawking once famously speculated that if a 'theory of everything' was ever achieved, 'then we would know the mind of God'.[14] It is safe to say this is a long way off. Nevertheless, theories may tell us something about how God makes things happen. In this vein, I want briefly to refer to quantum mechanics, where once again we find the conventions of space and time turned upside down.

Following on from the work of the physicists John Stewart Bell in the 1960s, and Stuart Freedman and John Clauser in the 1970s, Alain Aspect demonstrated experimentally in 1981 that a pair of photons first entangled and then sent off in different directions continue to react to each other instantaneously; if the spin of one photon is arrested, the other simultaneously stops. Photons have no charge and no mass. Being packets of electromagnetic energy (the stuff of light) they naturally travel at the speed of light. However, Aspect demonstrated that these

---

13. Shu (2010).
14. Hawking (1988: 175).

once-entangled photons were now communicating superluminally, that is, faster than the speed of light, demonstrating what is known as quantum non-locality.[15] It has since been confirmed that even the humble electron, which has both mass and a negative charge and which was thought to move at speeds less than the speed of light, spends more than half of its life in the superluminal state.

In 2012, the discovery of the Higgs boson hit the headlines.[16] Higgs bosons are constituents of the Higgs scalar field, which exists everywhere. Without the Higgs field, subatomic particles would simply ping around the universe forever at the speed of light and never form atoms and molecules. However, as these particles travel through the Higgs field, they acquire mass. Exactly how much mass depends on the particle in question. Peter Higgs and François Englert, who shared the Nobel Prize in 2013 for their discovery, have likened it to a snowfield: a bird can fly over it (photons); with skis you can glide across it (electrons); with snowshoes it takes more energy (quarks); and boots make for heavy going (W and Z bosons).

We may be looking at how the cosmos extends into multiple domains of space-time, our universe most probably being one such locale.[17] We should not really be surprised at this, for quantum non-locality shows us that time and space as we know them are merely local phenomena – hence the aphorism 'Time is what prevents everything from happening at once, and space is what prevents everything from happening to me!'[18]

The notion that life forms exist in a world of 'dead' matter is seriously out of date. On the contrary, all matter is 'alive'. The atoms that make up a piece of rock know how to organise themselves. The cells of a plant have the intelligence to turn the flower towards the sun. Animals have awareness like us. Human beings and a few other species with complex neurobiology, like dolphins, apes and elephants, show a further development: the awareness of being aware. Self-awareness is humanity's greatest evolutionary challenge, for not only does it bring us to the threshold of the transcendent, but it also gives us the power to destroy.

Since the transcendent cannot be measured, from the perspective of mainstream science it holds no interest. Yet quantum cosmology accommodates transcendent reality, since it argues that there is no objective world 'out there' that is independent of consciousness. The

---

15. Merali (2015).
16. CERN (n.d.).
17. It has been suggested that Jesus was alluding to this when he remarked: 'My Father's house has many rooms'. John 14:2. *The Holy Bible*, NIV.
18. Popularly attributed to the physicist John Archibald Wheeler.

observer and the observed cannot be separated. The quantum realm is non-causal, non-local and non-material. It only becomes causal, local and material with what is known as 'the collapse of the wave function', actuated by your consciousness, my consciousness and collectively, that of all humanity. What could be better suited to the transcendental perspective than partaking of a phenomenal world that materialises from a vibrant unitary field with majestic capacities greater than anything we can put into words?

Soul Awareness

Cosmologists who dare to think outside the box help to liberate us from the standoff between religion and material realism. From this vantage point, we can see that the spiritual impulse continues to well up like a stream flowing from deep underground, as shown by the demographic, 'spiritual but not religious'. As church attendance declines, the numbers in this unaligned group are rising, according to different surveys numbering somewhere between 15% and 45% of the population.[19]

Everyone has their own idea of what they mean by 'spirituality' and descriptions are wide-ranging.[20] They include: finding meaning and purpose in life; trusting that adversity can challenge us to grow and change; seeking wholeness of being; experiencing and expressing non-possessive, non-conditional love; readiness to forgive; recognising the oneness of all of life and working for its greater good; gratitude for the gift of life; searching for an understanding of birth, life and death within the compass of the infinite; and maintaining equanimity, courage, hope and acceptance in times of illness, loss and bereavement. Lastly, for many people, there is the felt presence of God.

I am using the word soul to convey the essence of individual human spirituality. The soul is a wellspring of unconditional love, forgiveness and healing and while it may be denied (and often is), it cannot be destroyed. As I understand it, while the soul knows its eternal home to be the non-material realm of the transcendent, it makes the human journey in order to help show us which path to take as we struggle through the challenges of life.

As a species, we are well endowed with intelligence, a rich emotional reality and the capacity to learn from experience. However, at

---

19. Survey by Theos (2013).
20. Also discussed in *Spirituality and Psychiatry – Crossing the Divide* and *Soul-Centred Psychotherapy*, both this volume.

this stage in the evolution of humankind, the ego is still geared to survival mentality along the lines of 'the more you have, the stronger you are'. Consequently, the ego identifies with personal possessions; hence the psychology of 'me' and 'mine'.[21] If there must be such a thing as the soul, the ego thinks of it as a kind of prized spiritual organ in its personal possession.

Yet when we engage with the faculty of the soul in reflection, prayer, contemplation or meditation, we realise to the contrary that the soul does not belong to us. Rather, we belong to it! When the ego is taken out of the equation, the personal boundaries we usually feel to be so important start to dissolve. Beyond the human drama playing out on the stage of the world, there is only the one soul, infinite and eternal, in which everything resides. Although we use words such as 'God' to name this boundless presence, such ultimate reality is beyond the reach of all language.

When we attune to the soul, the love that arises is the expression of the soul's own joy in being. This is very different to the emotional vagaries of the ego. While the ego needs to be loved, the soul desires to love. In fact, the soul enjoys nothing so much as 'acts of random kindness and senseless acts of beauty'.[22] To live estranged from the soul is a great misfortune.[23] Tell-tale signs of this impoverishment are restlessness, fatigue and depression. Restlessness arises from the painful emptiness that a person feels within, yet seeks to fill from without. Such is the beguiling nature of our consumer society that there are endless distractions for the ego to pursue. Nevertheless, when the search proves to be both fruitless and exhausting, depression not infrequently supervenes.

Importantly, depression can turn out to be the wake-up call that is so badly needed, alerting us to having lost touch with the soul and its purpose. When we acquiesce to the soul, we discover that our many fears – of failure, defeat, loneliness, loss, even death – are the anxious fixations of the ego. Just as a loving parent will reassure an anxious child, we can take the ego in hand and venture into the wider world, where the soul's purpose – to live not with fear but with love – can be put into practice.[24]

---

21. See also *Past Life Memory – A Key to Understanding the Self?*, this volume.
22. The Canadian author Anne Herbert first wrote these words on a placemat in Sausalito, California in 1982 as a reversal of the saying 'random acts of violence and senseless acts of cruelty'. Herbert (1995: 88).
23. Jesus points out, 'What good will it be for someone to gain the whole world, yet forfeit their soul?' Mark 8:36. *The Holy Bible*, NIV.
24. 'There is no fear in love. But perfect love drives out fear'. John 4:18. *The Holy Bible*, NIV.

In Conclusion

We are living at a pivotal time for the future of humanity, yet tragically the ego cannot comprehend what is at stake. The limitations of the ego can be likened to the story of the six blind men and the elephant. They each describe what they can feel with their hands – a wall, a tree, a rope and so on, but no one puts it together and comes up with the right answer.

This is why we need to pay attention to the soul. Human society today is geared to competition rather than collaboration, getting rich rather than having a sufficiency and winning the war while losing the peace. Yet the ego, although a slow learner, is not ineducable. With the right guidance it can be helped to give up its 'me or you' approach to survival in favour of 'me *and* you' – in other words 'we', as shown in this allegorical tale about heaven and hell. In hell, people are seated around a large dish of appetising food. They are obliged to use spoons with handles longer than their arms and since no one can get the spoon to the mouth, they are starving. In heaven, they must use the same spoons, but instead everyone sets about feeding each other.[25]

Our problem is that the human ego is still mired in its evolutionary past. If it is to have an evolutionary future, we must help it see that we are not just one species but one family sharing one home. Only then shall we make use of science wisely and well.

When the astronaut Edgar Mitchell beheld Earth, 'the blue planet', through the window of the spacecraft Apollo 14, he experienced a transformative awakening.[26] The vision of beauty and oneness inspired the remainder of his life's work with the message of unity. Fortunately, we do not need to go into outer space to have that same vision. We can appreciate it here and now by opening ourselves to the presence of the soul.

I am convinced that these most recent centuries we call modernity will turn out to be 'make or break' for humankind. From the thousands of millions of years this planet has existed and that have resulted in the evolution of *Homo sapiens*, in just a few decades we are going to find out whether humanity will survive and thrive, or whether we had our chance and missed it. How extraordinary to be born right now and what responsibility we bear!

I will end with one further reflection on heaven and hell. There is a rabbinical saying that goes like this: 'What is hell? It is when God

---

25. An allegory attributed to the Lithuanian preacher, Rabbi Haim of Romshishok.
26. Mitchell (2008).

sits you on his knee and shows you what your life could have been!' What about heaven? The rabbi does not say, so we will have to decide this for ourselves. According to the Gospel of Thomas, Jesus implored us not to live for tomorrow but for today. When asked 'On what day will the kingdom come?' Jesus answered, 'It will not come when it is expected. No one will say, "See, it is here!" or "Look, it is there!" But the Kingdom of the Father is spread over the earth and men do not see it'.[27]

We are being told not to wait for the day of reckoning but to act now. How then might we go about it? We do not have to look far, for the human ego, when taken in hand by the soul, becomes a perfect instrument for making heaven on Earth. If we could advance this one small step, it would be a giant leap for humankind.

References

Brierley Consultancy (2016) Christianity in the UK. Faith Survey. Available at: https://faithsurvey.co.uk/uk-christianity.html (accessed 8 July 2017).
Centre for Social Justice (2013) *Maxed Out: Serious Personal Debt in Britain*. CSJ. Available at: http://www.centreforsocialjustice.org.uk/library/maxed-serious-personal-debt-britain (accessed 8 July 2017).
CERN (n.d.) The Higgs boson. CERN. Available at: https://home.cern/topics/higgs-boson (accessed 8 July 2017).
Dawkins, R. (2007) *The God Delusion*. Black Swan.
Guo, X., Zheng, L., Wang, H., et al. (2013) Exposure to violence reduces empathetic responses to other's pain. *Brain and Cognition*, 82, 187–191.
Hawking, S. (1988) *A Brief History of Time*. Bantam Press.
Heller, M. (2009) *Ultimate Explanations of the Universe*. Springer.
Herbert, A. (1995) *Whole Earth Review*. Issue 85.
Laub, Z. (2016) The Islamic State. Council on Foreign Relations. Available at: http://www.cfr.org/iraq/islamic-state/p14811 (accessed 8 July 2017).
Merali, Z. (2015) Quantum 'spookiness' passes toughest test yet. *Nature*, 525, 14–15.
Meyer, M. & Bloom, H. (1993) *Gospel of Thomas* (Saying 113). Bravo.
Mitchell, E. (2008) *The Way of the Explorer: An Apollo Astronaut's Journey Through the Material and Mystical Worlds*. New Page Books.
Pew Research Center (2017) *The Changing Global Religious Landscape*. Available at: http://www.pewforum.org/2017/04/05/the-changing-global-religious-landscape/ (accessed 8 July 2017).
Sheldrake, R. (2012) *The Science Delusion*. Coronet.
Shu, W. (2010) The geometry of the universe. *Mathematics and Statistics*, 3, 75–88.
Theos (2013) *The Spirit of Things Unseen: Belief in Post-Religious Britain*. Theos. Available at: http://www.theosthinktank.co.uk/publications/2013/10/17/the-spirit-of-things-unseen-belief-in-post-religious-britain (accessed 8 July 2017).

---

27. Meyer & Bloom (1993).

16

Helping Patients Tell Their Story: Narratives of Body, Mind and Soul

In this paper, I aim to show that the narrative set in motion when a patient is seen by a psychiatrist is not only an account of an individual's life experience, but is also shaped by the expectations of the psychiatrist – more than either of them may be aware.

Gaining a clear understanding is especially relevant to soul narrative, which is often invested with profound personal meaning, yet can lead to confusion when not understood, or else is likely to remain unvoiced if a patient senses that their spiritual beliefs and concerns are not given credence. I will conclude by illustrating how the soul narrative, when encouraged, can bring real therapeutic benefits.

The Pre-eminence of Medical Diagnosis

In general medicine, taking a patient's history is followed by hands-on examination of the body, feeling for lumps and bumps, listening to the heart and lungs and testing for abnormalities of the nervous system, followed when needed by a battery of investigations. The unspoken contract between physician and patient enables doctors to divide their attention between relating to their patients as persons and yet examining their bodies with the detachment needed to identify pathology and arrive at an accurate diagnosis (in Greek, *dia* means 'stand apart', *gnosis* means 'discern').

The art of diagnosis has its roots in the ancient civilisations of Egypt, Greece and China. But the physician of our time is heir principally to a scientific method that began during the Renaissance with the

First published as chapter in *Spirituality and Narrative in Psychiatric Practice: Stories of Mind and Soul* (eds C.C.H. Cook, A. Powell & A. Sims), pp. 39–52. © 2016 The Royal College of Psychiatrists. Reproduced with permission.

study of human anatomy and that has brought extraordinary knowledge of how the body works. A correct diagnosis will generally indicate a disease that has recognisable pathology, a cause (aetiology), a natural history (it may progress or remit) and an outcome (prognosis). At best, getting the diagnosis right leads to a treatment that cures, and if not to cure, then at least to relief of symptoms or, when the condition is terminal, to quality end-of-life care.

Making the diagnosis requires a relentless kind of questioning impressed on every medical student and never forgotten: Where is the pain? Is it a dull ache or stabbing? Does it radiate? Does anything bring it on, or relieve it? How about exercise, or eating, or lying down? This kind of enquiry rapidly becomes second nature to doctors, like being a journalist on the trail of something suspicious and digging away until the whole picture emerges. The diagnostic narrative is relatively impersonal, focusing on the elucidation of physical symptoms and their causes. Yet general medicine has long had to take note of the body–mind connection. We know from liaison psychiatry and psychosomatic medicine that in-depth enquiry into a patient's personal life, feelings, stresses and habits may be required. Indeed, some 20% of patients in general practice present with underlying emotional disorder.[1] Common to all these consultations, however, is the straightforward aim of helping the patient back to physical health and well-being. If body and mind can be likened to car and driver, the driver is being questioned in order to help with getting the car back on the road.

Mental health science is likewise rooted in physical medicine. More than a century ago, abnormal states of mind secondary to nutritional diseases, syphilis, porphyria, hormonal disturbances and brain injury encouraged the search for physical causation. A minority of mental disorders are indeed secondary to organic pathology, as with endocrine disorders, neurodegenerative disease, or where there is a brain lesion. More recently, neurodevelopmental deficits have been implicated in a number of conditions, including autistic spectrum disorders and possibly schizophrenia. In the field of intellectual disability, genetic counselling and research are proving invaluable. These conditions highlight the importance of psychiatry as a branch of medicine and underline the value of the diagnostic narrative, even though it is uncommon in practice for a psychiatrist to come across an organic condition, except in the elderly.

---

1. De Waal et al. (2004).

Descriptive Psychopathology: A Two-edged Sword?

The broad acceptance of psychiatry as a medical specialty owes most to Emil Kraepelin's historic classification of the functional psychoses into schizophrenia and manic depression (bipolar disorder) at the end of the 19th century. Thereafter, it was thought to be only a matter of time before psychiatry would demonstrate the underlying biology of mental disorder. Yet to this day the aetiology of schizophrenia and bipolar disorder remain obscure. Neurochemical hypotheses having proved inconclusive, new hope is now being invested in brain studies in the search for definitive neuropathology.

The pressure is on, for while the prevalence of schizophrenia and bipolar disorder in the population has stayed the same at around 1–2% each, there now appears to be an epidemic of mental disorders. Some 25% of women and 12% of men will need treatment for depression in the course of a lifetime[2] and according to the World Health Organization, mental illness now affects one in ten adults, accounting for over 12% of the global burden of disease and over 30% of the total burden of disability.[3] Most of these conditions have no clear-cut aetiology and no consistent prognosis. The picture is often a complex interplay of constitutional, developmental and environmental factors coupled with situational stress.

Nevertheless, the diagnostic narrative in psychiatry, whether using the framework of the *International Classification of Diseases* (ICD) or of the *Diagnostic and Statistical Manual of Mental Disorders* (DSM), has been to attempt to define mental illness with the same objectivity and rigour as physical disorders. Yet for the most part, it has simply led to the categorisation of symptom clusters. Descriptive psychopathology usefully serves as the lingua franca among psychiatrists, but often has little to say about the cause (and outcome) of the presenting problem. Moreover, DSM and ICD between them encompass and label just about every aspect of the human condition. The questionable introduction in 1980 of the category of 'major depression' in DSM-III was followed by 21 million prescriptions for fluoxetine (Prozac) being dispensed over the next 10 years.[4] The global psycho-pharmaceutical industry currently makes annual profits of around 76 billion US dollars,[5]

---

2. Bridges (2014).
3. World Health Organization (2001). First discussed in *Whither the Soul of Psychiatry?*, this volume.
4. Shorter (2014).
5. Dewan (2014).

a powerful testament to the widespread appeal of the pharmaceutical narrative of mental disorder.[6]

Life Comes with a Health Warning

The indelicate quip, 'life is a sexually transmitted disease for which there is no treatment and which is uniformly fatal', pinpoints the reality of human suffering, something discussed by psychiatrists less than it deserves, possibly because we live in a culture that prefers a pharmaceutical narrative rather than facing up to the travails of humanity. How might we account for the soaring prevalence of mental disorder? Is the human race in decline? Is the world of materialism and consumerism eroding the core values that make life feel worthwhile?[7] Could it be, as Thomas Szasz suggested more than half a century ago, that the growing demographic of mental illness is symptomatic of a societal narrative that now habitually pathologises the human condition?[8]

These are complex matters and hard-pressed clinicians are not much given to questioning the extent that psychiatry mirrors an all-pervasive societal narrative. Nevertheless, most psychiatrists would agree that the continuum of distress extends from the pain of the human condition at the one end to severe (and often treatable) mental illness at the other.

However, a fundamental problem remains: much of psychiatry has been built on unsubstantiated premises for which no amount of classification can compensate.

Dynamic Psychopathology: Another Two-edged Sword?

All great institutions have to bear the strain of internal dissent. Psychiatry is no exception; a narrative competing with the biomedical model began more than a century ago with the work of Sigmund Freud. Freud promised a new understanding of the human mind in which doctor and patient would join in the search for meaning that lay encoded in the symptom; the symbolic life of the unconscious would be laid bare and its arcane mysteries revealed. For the first half of the 20th century, the narrative of psychoanalysis, known as 'the talking cure', reigned supreme in the Americas and Europe.

---

6. Davies (2013).
7. See *Modernity and the Beleaguered Soul*, this volume.
8. Szasz (1960).

Central to this narrative is the notion that the therapist listens to and interprets the unconscious significance of the patient's story. The understanding that follows relieves the patient of the symptom by revealing the source of emotions that have had to be repressed, denied or otherwise disavowed, as illustrated by the following example.

> Jean came into therapy with a history of recurrent panic attacks. The attacks intensified each time she entered into a serious relationship that might lead to an emotional commitment, yet she very much wanted to settle down and have a family. In therapy Jean suffered a severe panic attack during a session just before the summer break. With the help of the therapist, Jean was able to explore the significance of this panic, which brought back painful memories of childhood, when her mother had to be hospitalised for a lengthy period due to a life-threatening illness. Once Jean understood that her panic attacks were a resurgence of her fears of abandonment, the break could be successfully managed without further attacks. Three years after the conclusion of therapy, Jean wrote to let her therapist know she was now married and mother of a baby girl.

Countless people have benefited from such an approach. However, the outcome is not always successful and there has been ethical concern over the imbalance of power that arises. For instance, how can a patient give truly informed consent when the analysis of 'unconscious material' is the prerogative of the therapist? How free is the patient to disagree with the therapist when this can be interpreted as 'resistance'? What about the risk that the patient's narrative is being subtly appropriated by the therapist and re-fashioned according to the therapist's worldview? Seeing all of the human condition through the lens of dynamic psychopathology can result in therapy that is more a way of life than a treatment. Freud himself warned against this danger.[9]

Good therapists go to great lengths to avoid the abuse of power. Yet when a professional advises someone in need of help and who is less knowledgeable, the risk is always there, whether it be psychotherapy or pharmacotherapy. The more susceptible the patient, the greater the ethical obligation on the professional. Offering no conceptual map risks leaving the patient floundering, yet a favoured theoretical preconception can trammel a vulnerable mind.

If democracy of spirit is to prevail in the course of a psychological therapy, the therapist must take care not to make conjecture sound like fact (since no one can truly know what is in the mind of another), but rather to invite the patient to respond freely and authentically. No

---

9. Freud (1937).

matter how appealing and persuasive a theory may be, authenticity holds the key to genuinely therapeutic narrative. This has to be the touchstone if one's patient is going to find, in the telling, a new, creative and enduring meaning to their story.

Authentic Narrative

In an authentic exchange, the narrative is an act of co-creation. Authenticity requires that both people meet on the basis of equality as human beings, each contributing with their own experience. Therapeutic expertise is able to be valued and acknowledged, but it is important to recognise that 'therapist' and 'patient' are no more than complementary roles set up to enable the one to give to the other a special kind of assistance.

Across healthcare, the clinical setting favours the parent/child dynamic because of the knowingness of the clinician and the dependency needs of the patient. In some circumstances this is helpful, but there is the danger of precluding a more valid interpersonal exchange – validity founded on acknowledging that we are all travellers on life's journey, facing the same landmarks, losses, hopes and fears. As Carl Rogers remarked, 'what is most personal is most general'.[10] Without this awareness, no person, however clever and knowledgeable, could reach out and help another. Especially in mental healthcare, when this authority-based dynamic stands in the way of authenticity, the balance needs restoring. Then comes the discovery that each person is writing their own life story and that nobody can be the instrument for change except oneself.

The narrative that charts a person's life from birth through to this present moment must sooner or later find reconciliation with the past, for there is no changing the facts of the story, as the 10th-century Persian poet and philosopher Omar Khayyám wryly reflects:[11]

> 'The Moving Finger writes; and, having writ,
> Moves on: nor all thy Piety nor Wit
> Shall lure it back to cancel half a Line,
> Nor all thy Tears wash out a Word of it.'

What a person *can* change, however, is *how* to relate to those events of the past; whether to remain a victim of circumstance or to see adversity

---

10. Rogers (1961: 27).
11. Fitzgerald (1989).

as the grit that makes the pearl. The choice lies between repeating the same chapter over and over and starting a new one. Every story must have its past; the life-affirming story has a future too. When the ego, through force of habit, resists change, the clinician can invite a more soulful exchange to lend support, as will be described later.

The Power of Narrative for Good or Ill

A sign of mental health is that a person's chronicle of events and experiences forms a coherent and meaningful narrative; 'living' this narrative is an act of involuntary creativity that enriches the self and its circle of intimates. Some people reach a wider audience through the arts, education, business or politics. Not least, the great spiritual exemplars have touched innumerable lives with their uncompromising narratives of wisdom and truth. Of the spiritual teacher, the Zen scholar Daisetz Suzuki writes, 'His hands and feet are the brushes and the whole universe is the canvas on which he depicts his life… this picture is called history'.[12]

In contrast, psychotic narrative, while often vociferously proclaiming the 'truth', is likely to be painfully disjointed, or else tragically concrete, as in the case of a patient with schizophrenia convicted of homicide, who explained: 'I took a life because I needed one'.[13]

Groups, too, can spawn 'psychotic' narratives in which the individual is swept up by perverse ideology, resulting in horrific genocide as in Rwanda,[14] or mass suicide as in the case of the Jonestown massacre in Guyana,[15] when Jim Jones, the paranoid cult leader, commanded some 900 followers to take poison to 'save' them from the evils of the world.

On the other hand, surrender of the self to a higher power is a hallmark of religious belief. Speaking in tongues (the 'Toronto blessing') is endorsed by many evangelical Christians as a divine gift. Should such altered states of consciousness be regarded as psychopathological? Not necessarily, according to ICD-10, which under trance and possession disorder (F44.3) specifies: '…Include here only trance states that are involuntary or unwanted, occurring outside religious or culturally accepted situations'.[16] In this case, psychiatry must distinguish between mental illness and mental health solely on the context of the event.

---

12. Herrigel (1953: 8).
13. Cox (1982).
14. Ilibagiza (2006).
15. Scheeres (2011).
16. World Health Organization (2016).

Here we find a conflation of medical and social narratives that, while offering some practical help, does little to clarify what is really going on.

What, then, about people who join 'hearing voices' groups, in which many group members will have already been diagnosed as having mental illness? With the help of the group, a new kind of coherent narrative is established, based on sharing the experience of intrusive voices and how to challenge them and find ways to live with them. This may require strategies such as negotiating with the voices and insisting they wait until, say, the evening when they can be promised an hour of undivided attention.[17] Such narrative has moved away from the concept of psychopathology to becoming a means of adaptation. We might compare this with an amputee who, once the injury has been attended to, no longer regards himself as ill just because he will need a prosthesis.[18]

These various narratives illustrate that 'psychopathology' is context-bound and cannot be divorced from circumstance. Indeed, it is sometimes deemed necessary to detain and forcibly treat a person under the Mental Health Act. It can be especially hard to maintain any kind of constructive dialogue in these circumstances, for apart from the impact of the mental disorder itself, there is the further trauma of taking away a person's right to freedom, resulting in more confusion, fear and anger. The psychiatrist needs to be able to tolerate the outpouring of anger and distress by the patient while remaining 'present', being available and always ready to help make sense of the anguish and confusion as it passes.

The Spiritual Narrative

Psychiatrists face a unique challenge when evaluating experiences phenomenologically indistinguishable from mental illness, yet potentially invested with profound spiritual significance.[19] What distinguishes a person who has an acute and transient psychotic disorder from one who has what turns out to be a life-changing spiritual revelation? Consider this hallucinatory episode:[20]

---

17. Romme & Escher (1989).
18. See also *The Whole Patient*, this volume.
19. Lucas (2011).
20. A hallucination is defined as any percept-like experience which: (a) occurs in the absence of an appropriate stimulus, (b) has the full force or impact of the corresponding actual (real) perception, and (c) is not amenable to direct and voluntary control by the experiencer. World Health Organization (1992).

'As [Saul] neared Damascus on his journey, suddenly a light from heaven flashed around him. He fell to the ground and heard a voice saying to him, "Saul, Saul, why do you persecute me?" "Who are you, Lord?" Saul asked. "I am Jesus, whom you are persecuting", he replied [...] Saul got up from the ground, but when he opened his eyes he could see nothing. So they led him by the hand into Damascus. For three days he was blind, and did not eat or drink anything.

In Damascus there was a disciple named Ananias. [...] Placing his hands on Saul, he said, "Brother Saul, the Lord – Jesus, who appeared to you on the road as you were coming here – has sent me so that you may see again and be filled with the Holy Spirit." Immediately, something like scales fell from Saul's eyes, and he could see again.'[21]

Would Saul, later renamed Paul the Apostle, have been diagnosed today with acute and transient psychotic disorder (ATPD)? And what should we make of the risk of recurrence? Whereas many people who experience repeated episodes of ATPD never progress to chronic schizophrenia,[22] one in eight does so within 5 years.[23] Psychiatry has traditionally looked askance at spiritual and religious preoccupation because of this association with psychosis. Nevertheless, Harold Koenig[24] has demonstrated a broadly positive correlation between religion, spiritual practice and improved mental as well as physical health. Given that many people have such 'exceptional human experiences', leading them to a new sense of meaning and purpose in life, perhaps we should not too readily focus on psychopathology for fear that illness may lie ahead.

There continues to be controversy nonetheless. A study by Michael King[25] claims to show that religion confers no additional protection against mental disorder when compared with those people who are neither spiritual nor religious. King also unequivocally states that 'people who profess spiritual beliefs in the absence of a religious framework are more vulnerable to mental disorder'. While King does not go so far as to suggest that 'spirituality' causes mental disorder, it would be easy to draw that erroneous conclusion. There is, however, an important sociological perspective to consider. Contemporary Western society, with its erosion of deeper values and materialistic pursuit of pleasure, avoids asking difficult questions such as 'Why are we here?' and 'What it is all for?' If a person is deeply preoccupied with such existential concerns, they

---

21. Acts 9: 4, 5, 8–10, 17, 18. *The Holy Bible*, NIV.
22. Farooq (2012).
23. Queirazza et al. (2014).
24. Koenig et al. (2012).
25. King et al. (2013).

may well be labelled as depressed. Self-doubt and anguish have always been features of the spiritual life, as instanced by such historic persons as Julian of Norwich and John of the Cross. In the largely secular society of Britain today, there is a burgeoning demographic of 'spiritual but not religious', for whom soul-searching can be a lonely pursuit. Without a climate of understanding or the community support of a faith tradition, the individual seeker may well struggle. Kenneth Pargament points out that spiritual struggles have the potential for either good or bad mental health outcomes.[26] So, perhaps the question to ask is whether the world in which we now live is conducive to a good outcome.[27]

A more radical interpretation has been suggested by Russell Razzaque, who counters King's conclusion by suggesting that the finding is unremarkable, since people who have a mental disorder are more likely than others to be seeking a spiritual understanding of life. He writes: 'There is something at the core of the experience of mental illness that draws sufferers towards the spiritual. Their suffering is an echo of the suffering we all contain within us'.[28]

This issue comes to the fore when we consider how to respond to a person who is in need of psychiatric help and in the throes of a spiritual crisis, be it loss of faith or an experience of overwhelming spiritual significance. Mental health services provide little by way of spiritually informed care. Consequently, there is no way of knowing how often a transient psychotic episode might otherwise have become the turning point on a new path of meaning and purpose had the narrative only been explored in a different way.

This is a difficult area, especially as psychiatrists have a medically sanctioned role to relieve symptoms. Nor is it their job to proselytise, or to presume the role of spiritual advisor. Even so, by routinely taking a short spiritual history, serious misunderstandings can be avoided.[29] The Royal College of Psychiatrists has now affirmed that 'a tactful and sensitive exploration of patients' religious beliefs and spirituality should routinely be considered and will sometimes be an essential component of clinical assessment'.[30]

The discussion that takes place between patient and psychiatrist is potentially one of the most intimate the patient will ever have. Yet the more the narrative adheres to the medical diagnostic approach, the less will the dialogue engage with real existential concerns. Rather than

---

26. Pargament (2011).
27. Cook & Powell (2013).
28. Razzaque (2014: 5).
29. Eagger (2009).
30. Cook (2013: 10).

dive too deep, many psychiatrists argue that what appear to be tangled preoccupations with the self, the world and even the cosmos fade away on recovery, suggesting that the perplexity and ruminations were secondary to mental disorder – and are therefore best left well alone. At the same time, psychiatrists know that conflict, loss and soul-searching are implicated in most mental breakdowns. Body, mind and soul, whose interweaving remains the greatest conundrum in psychiatry, have to be taken together if the psychiatrist is to help the patient recover from breakdown to find wholeness of being.

Where Narratives of Science and Spirituality Meet

Classical science regards consciousness and its spiritual *essentia* (the soul) as epiphenomenal, arising from the physico-chemical processes of the brain. This approach, derived from Newtonian mechanics, treats the mind and its contents purely as emergent psychological phenomena (God included).

Such a physicalist approach is founded on study (and measurement) of the object. Because consciousness is experienced subjectively, it has therefore to be ruled out of court. Yet one thing everyone agrees on is that they are conscious! It seems that degrees of consciousness are present in all life forms, most probably in proportion to the complexity of neural structure. A cat or dog, for instance, has the sense of awareness similar to our own. But we humans have further evolved the capacity to be self-aware which, coupled with language, enables inner dialogue, personal history and identity, and freedom of choice.

The time-honoured metaphysical view, of which natural science has always been so intolerant, is now being reframed by the 'new' science of quantum field theory, which seeks to understand the experimentally proven non-local properties of consciousness.[31] This perspective regards consciousness as pre-existent and pre-eminent; the brain as the on-board computer taps into a ubiquitous field of consciousness, rather like a television picking up a broadcast signal, and integrates it with the memory store of each person's experiences. The result: a unique and personal self-aware narrative.

The implications of these two perspectives are very different. The physicalist view sees each human being as a discrete entity, having an inner world composed only of personal experience and communicating with others solely by means of the special sense organs. On this basis,

---

31. Hameroff & Chopra (2012).

rationalists argue that God is nothing but a mental projection, good for warding off the (ego's) fear of oblivion and death. The metaphysical view, on the other hand, sees every human being as participating in a shared consciousness that ultimately extends beyond the self, indeed beyond the bounds of individual birth and death. This approach is consonant with the proposition first made by Aristotle in *Metaphysics* that the whole is more than the sum of its parts; it opens the way to a fundamental figure/ground reversal so that 'God', far from being a mere projection, is the *materia prima* of all that is.

Must we choose either one or other narrative? Surely there is room for both, for the greater does not exclude the lesser. The physicist Thomas Campbell reminds us that the subsystem, in this case human intelligence, can never fully comprehend the system of which it is a part – what he calls the larger consciousness system.[32] Campbell uses the impartial language of physics when speaking of the data stream that conjoins part and whole. Yet in the subjective language of spirituality we find the same mystery in the powerful recognition that we belong to more than ourselves.[33]

The various faith traditions each frame this mystery in their own way. For example, while Islam deliberately refrains from representational images of Allah, the Judeo-Christian faiths envision God according to an archetypal Imago Dei. Hinduism has something of both; Brahman the supreme power cannot be described but manifests through a multitude of lesser deities. Buddhists eschew a personal God altogether, while the 'spiritual but not religious' demographic is more likely to speak of a unitive and all-embracing 'higher power' or 'ultimate truth'.

Narratives of the Soul

What, then, of the soul – a word notably absent from the vocabulary of psychiatry and strangely perhaps, given that psyche in Greek means soul? The soul does not have to imply transcendence; some will refer simply to what is best in humanity – compassion, wisdom, unconditional love and innate goodness. In this sense, everyone can be said to have a soul.

Others will regard the soul as the expression of the divine in human form – that we *are* souls and that this is the source of our capacity for love and our awareness of goodness, beauty and truth. To

---

32. Campbell (2007).
33. See also *Why Must We Suffer? A Psychiatrist Reflects*, this volume.

borrow from Pierre Teilhard de Chardin, the difference in perspective is whether we see ourselves as human beings on a spiritual journey or spiritual beings on a human journey.[34] Either way, the human soul escapes any narrow definition and yet it holds a sacred meaning for all creeds and cultures. As Carl Jung pointed out, the soul is an archetype with profound symbolism second only to the supreme archetype of the Imago Dei.[35]

From the standpoint of enabling their patients to come from the deepest place within, psychiatrists need to accept that words such as 'God' and 'soul' are for some people instinctive and necessary when questioning the meaning and purpose of human existence and what may lie beyond the physical bounds of birth and death. The psychiatrist simply needs to stay open-minded and be genuinely interested in where the spiritual narrative leads. The psychiatric assessment, not least the mental state examination, is necessarily structured and formal to a degree. Even so, once the patient's welfare and safety are assured and the necessary treatment measures are put in place, there is the opportunity for a different kind of heartfelt narrative to unfold. For the psychiatrist, this entails suspending judgement and engaging compassionately with one's patient as a fellow human being. It means being willing to 'accompany' the patient in searching for answers to the big questions of life and death, including the nature and purpose of the soul, while trusting that the mental health crisis, however painful, can lead to an enrichment of life and its values, sometimes with new and very different life goals.[36]

Much of this is what good counselling and psychotherapy offers – empathy, warmth and genuineness, as first researched 50 years ago.[37] But here the psychiatrist ventures further. Spirituality has two dimensions: the quest for answers to the ultimate meaning and purpose of life, and the experience of wholeness of being that can bring inner strength and peace. By supporting a soulful narrative, the psychiatrist helps those profound questions to be asked, perhaps for the first time.[38] Then, like the person who has been searching everywhere for their necklace until they realise it is already around their neck, the patient who begins to find their own answers to those deep questions

---

34. 'We are not human beings having a spiritual experience. We are spiritual beings having a human experience'. The saying has been attributed to both Teilhard de Chardin and G.I. Gurdjieff.
35. Jung (1959).
36. See *Soul-Centred Psychotherapy*, this volume.
37. Truax & Carkhuff (1967).
38. Royal College of Psychiatrists (2014).

discovers a wisdom they never knew they had and that can help bring peace of mind.

Such conversations are, in fact, conversations 'soul-to-soul'. Whatever arises happens naturally and exactly as it should, when the psychiatrist is able to be fully 'present' and concerned only to help the patient find their 'truth'.

The soul narrative can often be elicited with a few simple prompts. Sometimes it helps to amplify what a patient has begun to say or to encourage a person to think the 'unthinkable'. For instance, if someone is contemplating suicide, it is worth finding out whether they believe death is the absolute and final end. If the patient is unsure (as many are), it makes sense to ask 'If there were to be an existence or a world beyond, how would you imagine it to be?' Encouragement to step outside the life being lived can bring a different perspective to bear, one that is wiser, more forgiving and more compassionate than the harsh self-judgement that so often accompanies mental anguish, as the following example shows:

> A young man burdened with a deep sense of failure and unable to see any future spoke of finding himself in fear and trembling before God. Invited by the therapist to 'listen' to what God might say to him, to his surprise he found himself being gently admonished, then lovingly told to continue with his life and to remember that success is not measured by wealth or fame but by finding love for his friends, his family and himself.

In cases of traumatic bereavement, the psychiatrist can ask about things left unresolved or unsaid that might be important to address. Often the patient will begin by saying it is too late. Instead, they can be invited to close their eyes, form a picture of the loved one and speak to them as if they were right there in the room. Not only can what was unexpressed now be voiced, but a narrative of healing can begin. By guiding the patient into a conversation (e.g. 'What do you need to ask/tell the person?' followed by 'Now listen to what they need to say to you') the soul can make itself heard, as shown in this example:

> A middle-aged woman had cared for her ageing father during his final illness and decline. Although close, their relationship had often been a tense one, and as he became more infirm and fought his disability, she often felt he was fighting her too. At times she got frustrated and angry, and then guilty for having such feelings. After her father passed away, she became depressed, reproaching herself for not 'having done better'. Assisted by the psychiatrist, she was able to 'meet' her father. She was encouraged to tell him about feeling how she had let him down. To her surprise, the answer came back that he was deeply grateful for the help and support she had given. He 'said' to her, 'I know you did your very

best. I am grateful, I love you and I want you to be happy'. The daughter and father could now part with a loving farewell.

Often problems that might seem insoluble can be approached by 'going within' and listening to the soul directly:

> A man brought up alone by an abusive, alcoholic mother was suffering from chronic depression, heavily laced with anger towards his mother. He could see that bitterness was spoiling his life but could only bring himself to say 'I'll never forgive what she did to me'. The therapist asked him if he wished that he could forgive. He replied, 'more than anything but it's impossible'. The psychiatrist now knew that although the egoic mind would not relent, the soul's capacity for forgiveness was present, so she invited him to 'go within' and find out what his heart would say if it could only speak.[39] His heart said to him, 'I am in such pain. All this anger is hurting me. Please stop before I break. I'm here to bring love into your life. Don't turn your back on me'. The patient fell silent for a while, sighed and then said, to himself as much as the psychiatrist, 'It's time I stopped hating and started loving. I want to get a life while there's time'.

In Conclusion

I have set out to show how, across a wide range of clinical objectives, paying attention to narrative is important both for diagnosis and for treatment. Starting from the physical, I describe how the narrative changes when engaging with the mental, and how making sense of the patient's story becomes a co-creation of doctor and patient. Lastly, I explore how narrative changes yet again when the focus moves to the spiritual.

This further shift is a profound one, for the narrative of the soul knows no bounds. Transcending the limitations of the mundane life, soul wisdom brings a deeper understanding to the human predicament. When the psychiatrist is willing to be fully 'present', and is able to offer a genuine and heartfelt connection to the individual who is in pain, the way is opened to reconciliation, forgiveness and peace of mind. The key lies in this: although the ego may be deeply aggrieved, the soul always seeks to love. The psychiatrist who can reach out to the soul in their patient is privileged to share in a narrative that brings healing to the psyche and fresh hope to the dispirited.

---

39. Cf. *Le cœur a ses raisons, que la raison ne connait point* ('The heart has its reasons, which reason does not know'). Pascal (1660). In Trotter (2005: 277).

References

Bridges, S. (2014) Mental health problems. In *Health Survey for England 2014*. Health and Social Care Information Centre. Available at: http://healthsurvey.hscic.gov.uk/support-guidance/public-health/health-survey-for-england-2014/mental-health-problems.aspx (accessed 8 July 2017).

Campbell, T. (2007) *My Big Toe: A Trilogy Unifying Philosophy, Physics, and Metaphysics: Awakening, Discovery, Inner Workings*. Lightning Strike Books.

Cook, C.C.H. (2013) *Recommendations for Psychiatrists on Spirituality and Religion* (Position Statement PS03/2013). Royal College of Psychiatrists.

Cook, C.C.H. & Powell, A. (2013) Spirituality is not bad for our mental health. *British Journal of Psychiatry*, 202, 385–386.

Cox, M. (1982) 'I took a life because I needed one': psychotherapeutic possibilities with the schizophrenic offender-patient. *Psychotherapy and Psychosomatics*, 37, 96–105.

Davies, J. (2013) *Cracked: Why Psychiatry is Doing More Harm Than Good*. Icon Books.

De Waal, M., Arnold, I., Eekhof, J., et al. (2004) Somatoform disorders in general practice: prevalence, functional impairment and comorbidity with anxiety and depressive disorders. *British Journal of Psychiatry*, 184, 470–476.

Dewan, S.S. (2014) *Drugs for Treating Mental Disorders: Technologies and Global Markets* (BCC Market Research Report PHM074B). BCC Market Research.

Eagger, S. (2009) *A Guide to the Assessment of Spiritual Concerns in Mental Healthcare*. RCPsych SPSIG. Available at: www.rcpsych.ac.uk/spsigarchive

Farooq, S. (2012) Is acute and transient psychotic disorder (ATPD) mini schizophrenia? The evidence from phenomenology and epidemiology. *Psychiatria Danubina*, 24 (suppl. 3), 311–315.

Fitzgerald, E. (1989) (transl.) *The Rubáiyát of Omar Khayyám*. Collins.

Freud, S. (1937) Analysis terminable and interminable. Reprinted [1968] in *The Standard Edition of the Complete Psychological Works of Sigmund Freud*, vol. 23. Hogarth Press.

Hameroff, S. & Chopra, D. (2012) The 'quantum soul'. In *Exploring Frontiers of the Mind-Brain Relationship* (eds A. Moreira-Almeida & F. Santana Santos). Springer.

Herrigel, E. (1953) *Zen in the Art of Archery*. Routledge and Kegan Paul.

Ilibagiza, I. (2006) *Left To Tell*. Hay House.

Jung, C. (1959) Researches into the phenomenology of the self. In *C.G. Jung: The Collected Works*, vol. 9, part 2: Aion. Routledge and Kegan Paul.

King M., Marston L., McManus S., et al. (2013) Religion, spirituality and mental health: results from a national study of English households. *British Journal of Psychiatry*, 202, 68–73.

Koenig, H.G., King, D.E. & Carson, V.B. (2012) *Handbook of Religion and Health*, 2nd edn. Oxford University Press.

Lucas, C. (2011) *In Case of Spiritual Emergency*. Findhorn Press.

Pargament, K.I. (2011) *Spiritually Integrated Psychotherapy: Understanding and Addressing the Sacred*. Guilford Press.

Queirazza, F., Semple, D.M. & Lawrie, S.M. (2014) Transition to schizophrenia in acute and transient psychotic disorders. *British Journal of Psychiatry*, 204, 299–305.

Razzaque, R. (2014) *Breaking Down is Waking Up*. Watkins Publishing.

Rogers, C. (1961) *On Becoming a Person: A Therapist's View of Psychotherapy*. Houghton Mifflin.

Romme, M. & Escher, A. (1989) Hearing voices. *Schizophrenia Bulletin*, 15, 209–216.

Royal College of Psychiatrists (2014) Spirituality and mental health. RCPsych. Available at http://www.rcpsych.ac.uk/mentalhealthinformation/therapies/spiritualityandmentalhealth.aspx (accessed 3 July 2017).

Scheeres, J. (2011) *A Thousand Lives: The Untold Story of Jonestown*. Simon & Schuster.

Shorter, E. (2014) The 25th anniversary of the launch of Prozac gives pause for thought: where did we go wrong? *British Journal of Psychiatry*, 204, 331–332.

Szasz, T. (1960) The myth of mental illness. *American Psychologist*, 15, 113–118.

Trotter, W.F. (transl.) (2005) *Blaise Pascal: Pensées (Thoughts)*. Section IV: 'Of the Means of Belief'. Digireads.com.

Truax, C.B. & Carkhuff, R.R. (1967) *Towards Effective Counseling and Psychotherapy*. Aldine.

World Health Organization (1992) *International Statistical Classification of Diseases and Related Health Problems, 10th Revision* (ICD-10). WHO.

World Health Organization (2001) *Mental Health – A Call for Action by World Health Ministers* (World Health Report). WHO.

World Health Organization (2016) *International Statistical Classification of Diseases and Related Health Problems, 10th Revision* (ICD-10), Version: 2016. WHO. Available at: http://apps.who.int/classifications/icd10/browse/2016/en (accessed 3 July 2017).

17

Prejudice – Can We Live Without It?

The subject of prejudice does not feature, as far as I know, on the curriculum for psychiatrists in training. Nor, I suspect, does it appear in the learning objectives for other mental health professionals. I had not given it much thought either before being invited to speak on the subject, so my contribution cannot be counted as expert in any way. However, I have found the required preparation personally fruitful and I hope others, too, will find the question worthy of consideration.

I would like to start with this well-known Zen story:

> The Zen master Hakuin was praised by his neighbours for living a pure life. A beautiful Japanese girl, whose parents owned a food store, lived nearby. Suddenly, without any warning, her parents discovered she was with child. She would not confess who the man was, but after much harassment at last named Hakuin.
>
> In great anger the parents went to the master. 'Is that so?' was all he would say.
>
> After the child was born it was brought to Hakuin. By this time he had lost his reputation, which did not trouble him, but he took very good care of the child. He obtained milk from his neighbours and everything else he needed.
>
> A year later the girl's mother could stand it no longer and she told her parents the truth that the real father of the child was a young man who worked in the fish market. The mother and father of the girl at once went to Hakuin to ask forgiveness, to apologise at length, and to get the child back.
>
> Hakuin was willing. In yielding the child, all he said was: 'Is that so?'

How many of us could lose our reputation and good name and retain complete equanimity in the face of such undeserved prejudice?

Paper prepared for conference 'Silent Prejudice, Stigma and Spirituality', held by the Spirituality and Psychiatry Special Interest Group at the Royal College of Psychiatrists, London, April 2017.

Now for a story of my own: one hot summer day in 1981, rioting broke out in the predominantly Black neighbourhood of Brixton, London. My home was close by and from the garden I could see billowing smoke and flames. The air reverberated with the noise of breaking glass, screams and police sirens. On the radio, I heard that rioters were on the march and would be coming past my house. Immediately I rushed about looking for a weapon to defend my home and young family. I found an axe and waited inside the front door, prepared for the worst. As it happened, the rioters took a different route, but this was a great lesson to me. I had seen myself as a tolerant, liberal-minded psychiatrist and within a few minutes, I had become capable of extreme violence.

It could be argued that defending one's family is a natural instinct. Yet there was something else that I was forced to admit – the world had suddenly become a place of 'us' and 'them', us being the peaceable, White, home-owning professional class and them being the angry and dispossessed Black community living a few streets away. Feeling acutely threatened, my prejudice had taken me by storm.

As widely used, 'prejudice' means a preconceived opinion that is not based either on reason or on actual experience – a negative prejudgement about a group or its members.[1] More than just a statement of opinion or belief, prejudice is imbued with feelings such as contempt or even loathing. Paradoxically, in its extreme form it can result in sheer indifference to the fate of one's fellow human being, for instance, as shown by the treatment of the Jews and others in Hitler's death camps. Indifference arises when a person is no longer seen as a human being. We see such dehumanisation today in what is called 'the war against terror', in which neither side views the other as remotely deserving of compassion.

In trying to account for prejudice, social scientists have looked at how we make judgements. Gordon Allport points out that 'the human mind must think with the aid of categories… Once formed, categories are the basis for normal prejudgment. We cannot possibly avoid this process. Orderly living depends upon it'.[2]

While categories are seemingly clear cut, they are in fact only approximations.[3] For example, there is a continuum between good and

---

1. The word prejudice first appears in the English language in the 14th century. Its etymology is from the Latin *prae* (meaning 'in advance') and *judicium* ('judgement'). There is an assumption also of unfairness, the Latin *praejudicium* meaning 'injustice'.
2. Allport (1979: 20).
3. Plous (2003).

evil, summer and winter flow one into the other, and the male and female genders, too, are blurred these days. Categories may help us read the map but the map is not the territory. In the case of prejudice, categorising turns into categorical thinking that distorts perception. Differences between the in-group and out-group are exaggerated while intra-group heterogeneity is glossed over. This leads to stereotyping. Even children under 3 years of age will stereotype, as shown by one study of anti-Arab prejudice in Israeli infants.[4] Tragically, such stereotypes are self-perpetuating unless vigorously countered.

Here is a shortlist of the devastating effects of prejudice: racism, including White supremacism and slavery; anti-Semitism and Islamophobia; religious war, genocide and so-called 'ethnic cleansing'; stereotyping and stigmatisation; class and status elitism; sexism and gender oppression; and (in youth-driven societies) ageism. To this I would add the subtle but pervasive prejudice of scientism.[5]

I now want to turn to early human history in suggesting that prejudice has been around a very long time.

The first advanced hominid was *Homo neanderthalensis*, a skilled tool maker who provided care and shelter for his family group. Neanderthals lived a nomadic life, with ample territory for hunting across Europe and Russia, and it is thought internecine feuding was rare – the enemy primarily was the cold climate. Then *Homo sapiens* came out of Africa around 200,000 years ago. Migrating across Asia and Europe, *Homo sapiens* overlapped with the Neanderthals and we know some interbreeding took place.[6] However, about 40,000 years ago, Neanderthals became extinct. Why this happened remains something of a mystery but at the very least, *Homo sapiens* had the advantage of a larynx better suited to the development of speech, and seem to have outstripped the Neanderthal in cultural complexity and the capacity for symbolisation.[7]

The Neolithic age, beginning around 10,000 years ago, marked the worldwide migration of *Homo sapiens*. Human society now took a

---

4. Bar-Tal (1996).
5. The Spirituality and Psychiatry Special Interest Group, while valuing science, rejects scientism as a narrow and limiting perspective on reality. See also *Modernity and the Beleaguered Soul*, this volume.
6. Up to 4% of Neanderthal genomic material is present in non-African people today. See Kuhlwilm et al. (2016).
7. There may also have been genetic differences of temperament comparable with the two species of great apes living today, chimpanzees and bonobos. In contrast to the chimpanzee, the bonobo is exceptionally peace loving and as a result, bonobos have become an endangered species.

giant step towards culturalisation with the development of agriculture, husbandry, property, advanced tool-making and a progressively structured, hierarchical social order. It is very likely that this also marks the era when endemic conflict among humans first arose – since when it has never stopped.

The increasing complexity of human society and the civilisations that arose are testimony to the power of the human ego in driving forward the human species' mastery over the animal kingdom and the natural world. However, all has not gone well subsequently with the balance of Nature.[8]

In the Neolithic era, *Homo sapiens* numbered around 1 million, increasing to 1 billion 200 years ago, 3 billion by 1960 and today 7.5 billion. At the same time, increasing numbers of human beings are being killed by their own kind.[9] The animal kingdom is not being spared either. Countless animal species have been eliminated; since 1900, the animal kingdom has suffered around 1000 times the natural background extinction rate (known as the sixth mass extinction in Earth's history). Meanwhile, the destruction inflicted on the planet – on its atmosphere, hydrosphere, cryosphere, geosphere and biosphere – looks set to result in a global catastrophe in our children's lifetime if not our own.[10]

Is there anything psychiatry might have to say about the apparently suicidal behaviour of the human species? Let us start with a simple medical analogy – that of autoimmune disease. We depend for our survival on antibodies that develop in response to an otherwise lethal array of antigens, viral, bacterial and chemical. However, when the immune system goes into overdrive and attacks the self, the consequences can be dire. So it is with the psychological defence mechanisms that

---

8. In the story of Creation, God blesses humankind with these words: 'Be fruitful and increase in number; fill the earth and subdue it. Rule over the fish in the sea and the birds in the sky and over every living creature that moves on the ground' (Genesis 1:28. *The Holy Bible*, NIV.) Whether or not we take the story of creation literally, this was an extraordinarily prescient depiction of what later was to come, although not, unfortunately, in the benign form of stewardship intended. *Homo sapiens* has instead appropriated the Earth for its own purposes, showing none of the forethought and humility that would have been needed to ensure that the species remained in balance and harmony with the abundance of Creation.
9. Excessive population density and its social consequences may be contributing to this. Cf. studies of rodent ethology, showing that overcrowding (of rats) leads to uncontrollable aggression that can result in decimation of the colony. Calhoun (1962).
10. See also *Technology and Soul in the 21ˢᵗ Century*, this volume.

determine how we respond psychologically to threat. In earlier human civilisations, these mechanisms ensured group survival, yet today the same defences threaten us with destruction. We can understand this better by taking a look at the propensities of the human ego.

The ego is an indispensable function of the psyche. It is the means by which a child becomes conscious of its identity – indeed, that it exists as a 'self'. For this to happen, the ego first enables the child to learn the difference between 'me' and 'not me'. The distinction between awareness of self and other gives each of us a mind of our own, a unique admixture of thoughts and feelings, with a personal narrative that weaves us into a timeline of past, present and future.

The ego drives the child to explore the world with curiosity and a sense of adventure. With socialising comes the discovery of group kinship and the cultural richness of all that follows. However, what I want to highlight here is that self-awareness greatly complicates what it means to be a social animal. I will illustrate briefly with reference to the model of the 'triune brain', put forward by Paul MacLean over 50 years ago.[11]

The so-called 'reptilian brain' includes the basal ganglia and structures derived from the floor of the forebrain. MacLean argued that it is responsible for behaviours involved in aggression, dominance and territoriality.[12] The 'paleomammalian brain' comprises the nuclei of the limbic system, which MacLean saw as governing motivation and emotion involved in feeding, reproductive and parental behaviour. Last but not least, there is the 'neomammalian brain' or cerebral neocortex, the most recent stage in evolution, conferring the ability for language, symbolisation, abstraction, planning, perception and, crucially, empathy. When humans feel safe from threat and sustained by loving relationships, there is harmonious integration of these three levels of functioning, resulting in adaptive and mature human behaviour. Nevertheless, this is a fragile balance and stress unmasks more primitive behaviour.

To come back to my story of the Brixton riots; as my anxiety soared, my adrenaline-charged limbic brain went into overdrive and in that moment I might have killed.[13] As soon as I calmed down, the humanitarian values of my upbringing (and profession) reasserted themselves, and the wave of prejudice subsided as quickly as it had

---

11. Many neuroscientists today regard the model as simplistic, for example, LeDoux (2012). Nevertheless, the model of the triune brain provides a useful schema of our evolutionary heritage.
12. For a detailed study, see Naumann (2015).
13. Although we are conditioned to resist such impulses, this mode of function is sanctioned in warfare and medals are awarded.

arisen. I was very much aware, however, that had my childhood been different, I may have been left with my prejudices reinforced, since past experiences shape our response to threats real or imagined, and generally it is belief, not fact that wins the day. It has been said that if you give a person a gun, that person may kill dozens, but if you give a person an ideology, that person may kill countless thousands.

How might we better understand the unconscious dynamics of prejudice? Psychoanalysis has something very useful to say here about ego defences. Children who live in fear of abandonment cannot risk getting angry with their parents or caregivers. Anger is associated with vulnerability and must therefore be got rid of. If this can be achieved, then the threat is gone both outwardly (the needed caregiver will not retaliate) and inwardly (the ego is now free from contamination with anger, and so can hope to be lovable). Nevertheless, the split-off anger needs to go somewhere and so it gets projected into a suitably vulnerable 'other', where it can be treated with contempt, attacked and (in accordance with magical thinking) destroyed.[14] This dynamic of splitting and projection characterises scapegoating and abusive relationships in particular, but it also applies to human society more widely,[15] as I shall be describing.

Carl Jung was well aware of the destructive side of human nature. He observed that the 'persona' we show the world serves to conceal the 'shadow' aspect of the self.[16] Jung's concern was to make the shadow conscious, not only to confront the ego with its blind conceit, but also to disarm the shadow of its destructive power by containing it and valuing it as part of the self. Both psychoanalysis and Jungian psychology envisage health as freedom from distortion of reality due to unconscious projections.[17]

I drew attention earlier to the emerging social complexity that defined the onset of the Neolithic era. *Homo sapiens* evolved a group culture that allowed for differentiation of labour, better provision for care of the young, a milieu in which bonding of kith and kin could be established, and more effective protection of the species when under threat. As agrarian communities enlarged, control moved from the family to centres of influence and power. Politics was born in the form of fiefdoms, nepotism and, of course, taxes.

---

14. Klein (1957).
15. See also *Psychosocial Implications of the Shadow*, in Powell (2017).
16. Jung (1959).
17. For Jung, this is ultimately the business of the soul, as revealed posthumously in the *Red Book*, a record of his private reflections written in the period 1915–1930 and finally made public in 2009 (Jung, 2012).

Sigmund Freud has described how the group leader carries the ego ideal for the group.[18] At best, this is a force for good but at worst, it renders the group susceptible to manipulation, such as we see in the politics of extreme nationalism and religious fundamentalism.[19] Such movements are generally accompanied by suppression of individual freedoms in favour of a rigidly imposed and unquestioned group norm.[20]

At times of conflict and unrest, group mechanisms of defence come into play. The state, the military and state-sanctioned religions strengthen social cohesion by means of splitting and projection (it is well known that a nation is never more united than when at war). All war, whether political, territorial, ethnic or religious, is centred on an ego ideal that justifies the need to fight: in order to proselytise (the truth must be imposed if resisted), to defend against incursion (the right of sovereignty), to regain what was once taken (righting a historical wrong), to claim territory (the 'just' appropriation of assets) or to unify the group (when in danger of fragmenting). This last manoeuvre is a device by means of which a leadership in danger of being overthrown creates an enemy and thereby preserves its power. [21]

I am alluding here to the broad sweep of nation states, but, like a fractal that repeats over and over, we find the same mechanisms at work in sectarian disputes, in local communities where there is ethnic and cultural division and in troubled families, for more than anything, war is a state of mind.[22]

In summary, prejudice is a persistent derogatory attitude based on a separative ego mentality that dissociates self from other. Rooted in fear, although often masked by compensatory grandiosity, it seeks to find fault with the alien 'other' rather than engage in honest self-examination.[23] When a group holds a prejudice, cohesion is strengthened

---

18. Freud (1921).
19. As described in Aldous Huxley's novel *Brave New World*, which portrays a benign but soulless tyranny. Huxley (2007).
20. Democratic societies are not always exempt as people suppose. Much 'conspiracy theory' is based on the supposition that while freedom of expression is permitted so that people can feel they have a voice, the real power-broking continues unabated, unaccountable and hidden from scrutiny.
21. George Orwell's futuristic novel *Nineteen Eighty-Four* powerfully portrays such a dystopia. Orwell (1949).
22. Individual patients may attend with a psychiatric label because they are unwittingly carrying the split-off projections of their partner or family, in which case attempting to treat the patient in isolation only serves to reinforce pre-existing dynamics.
23. Hence the saying of Jesus in defence of the woman accused of adultery: 'Let any

but at the cost of the groups' humanity. Splitting and projection blunt the capacity of the psyche to see the whole picture. Instead, group self-esteem is narcissistically reinforced by its intolerance of difference.

The ego's protective stance inclines people to seek out similarities of educational attainment, political affiliation, religious beliefs, social habits, sexual orientation and much more besides. Yet what we find in today's multicultural world is a bewildering array of differences – of skin colour, dress, language, religion, social attitudes and much more besides. The insecure ego is all too quick both to offend and to take offence, in consequence spending a good deal of its time on the brink of outrage.

What is to be done? Rather than get caught up in these perturbations, we can be guided by the soul, the spiritual birthright of every human being. On the mundane level, personal differences will always be visible since we are uniquely made. Yet when we go beyond the appearance of things, we discover the unbroken wholeness from which all life arises, from which it follows that self and other are as inseparable as two sides of one coin.

This is how the soul understands it to be. Unmoved by the prejudices of the ego, the soul persists in loving indiscriminately and unconditionally. Where fear is divisive, love is unitive; where fear is separation, love is connection; where fear is constraint, love is freedom; where fear says 'mine', love says 'ours'.

Allport, in the language of the social sciences, gives the following advice:

> 'Prejudice… may be reduced by equal status contact between majority and minority groups in the pursuit of common goals. The effect is greatly enhanced if this contact is sanctioned by institutional supports… and provided it is of a sort that leads to the perception of common interests and common humanity between members of the two groups'.[24]

This all makes good sense, yet it does not move the heart. Instead, I will end with a story told by the late Aikido master Terry Dobson, who describes a turning point in his life, one day on a train in the suburbs of Tokyo:[25]

> 'At one station the doors opened and a man bellowing at the top of his lungs shattered the quiet afternoon, yelling violent, obscene curses, staggered into our carriage. He was big, drunk and dirty. Screaming, he

---

    one of you who is without sin be the first to throw a stone' (John 8:7. *The Holy Bible*, NIV).
24. Allport (1979: 281).
25. An abridged passage from *A Kind Word Turneth away Wrath*. Dobson (1995: 153–156).

swung at the first person he saw, a woman holding a baby. The blow glanced off her shoulder, sending her spinning into the laps of an elderly couple. It was a miracle that the baby was unharmed.

The passengers were frozen with fear. I stood up. I was young and I'd been putting in a solid eight hours of Aikido training every day for the past three years. "This is it!" I said to myself as I got to my feet. "People are in danger. If I don't do something fast, somebody will probably get hurt."

Seeing me stand up, the drunk saw a chance to focus his rage. I wanted him mad because the madder he got, the more certain my victory. I blew him a sneering, insolent kiss. It hit him like a slap in the face. He gathered himself for a rush at me.

A split-second before he moved, someone shouted "Hey!" It was ear splitting. I remember being hit by the strangely joyous, lilting quality of it. "Hey!" We both stared down at a little old Japanese man. He took no notice of me, but beamed delightedly at the drunk, as though he had a most important, most welcome secret to share. "Come here," the old man said, "Come here and talk with me." He waved his hand lightly. "Talk to you," the drunk roared, "Why the hell should I talk to you?" The old man continued to beam at him without a trace of fear or resentment. "What'ya been drinking?" he asked lightly, his eyes sparkling with interest. "I been drinking sake and it's none of your goddam business". "Oh, that's wonderful," the old man said with delight, "I love sake too. Every night, me and my wife (she's 76, you know), we warm up a little bottle of sake and take it out into the garden, and we sit on the old wooden bench and watch the sun go down, and we look to see how our persimmon tree is doing. My grandfather planted that tree, you know, and we worry about whether it will recover from those ice-storms we had last winter. Persimmons do not do well after ice-storms, although I must say that ours has done rather better than I expected, especially when you consider the poor quality of the soil. Still, it is most gratifying to watch when we take our sake and go out to enjoy the evening – even when it rains!" He looked up at the drunk, eyes twinkling, happy to share his delightful information.

As he struggled to follow the old man's conversation, the drunk's face began to soften. His fists slowly unclenched. "Yeah," he said slowly, "I love persimmons, too…" His voice trailed off. "Yes", said the old man, smiling, "and I'm sure you have a wonderful wife."

"No" replied the drunk, "my wife died." He hung his head. Very gently, swaying with the motion of the train, the big man began to sob. "I got no wife, I got no home, I got no job, I got no money, I got nowhere to go. I'm so ashamed of myself." Tears rolled down his cheeks and a spasm of pure despair rippled through his body. Just then, the train arrived at my stop. As the doors opened I heard the old man cluck sympathetically. "My, my," he said, "That is a very difficult predicament, indeed. Sit down here and tell me about it."

I turned my head for one last look. The drunk was sprawled on the seat, his head in the old man's lap. The old man was softly stroking the filthy, matted head.

As the train pulled away, I sat down on a bench. What I had wanted to do with muscle and meanness had been accomplished with a few kind words. I had just seen Aikido tried in combat, and the essence of it was love.'

Returning to the title of this paper, 'Prejudice – can we live without it?', my answer is yes, we must, if there is to be a future for humanity.

References

Allport, G.W. (1979) *The Nature of Prejudice*. Basic Books.
Bar-Tal, D. (1996) Development of social categories and stereotypes in early childhood: the case of 'the Arab' concept formation, stereotype and attitudes by Jewish children in Israel. *International Journal of Intercultural Relations*, 20, 341–370.
Calhoun, J.B. (1962) Population density and social pathology. *Scientific American*, 206, 139–148.
Dawkins, R. (1976) *The Selfish Gene*. Oxford University Press.
Dobson, T. (1995) A kind word turneth away wrath. In *The Awakened Warrior* (ed. R. Fields). Tarcher/Putnam.
Freud, S. (1921) Group psychology and the analysis of the ego. Reprinted [1955] in *The Standard Edition of the Complete Psychological Works of Sigmund Freud*, vol. 18 (trans. & ed. J. Strachey). Hogarth Press.
Huxley, A. (2007) *Brave New World*. Vintage Classics.
Jung, C.G. (1959) Archetypes of the collective unconscious. In *C.G. Jung: The Collected Works*, vol. 9, part 1: The Archetypes and The Collective Unconscious (eds H. Read, M. Fordham & G. Adler). Routledge and Kegan Paul.
Jung, C.G. (2012) *The Red Book (Liber Novus)*. W.W. Norton.
Klein, M. (1957) *Contributions to Psycho-analysis*. Hogarth Press.
Kuhlwilm, M., Gronau, M., Hubisz, C., et al. (2016). Evidence mounts for interbreeding bonanza in ancient human species. *Nature*, 530, 429–433.
LeDoux, J. (2012) Evolution of human emotion: a view through fear. *Progress in Brain Research*, 195, 431–442.
Naumann, R. (2015) The reptilian brain. *Current Biology*, 25, 317–321.
Orwell, G. (1949) *Nineteen Eighty-Four*. Penguin Classics.
Plous, S. (2003) The psychology of prejudice, stereotyping, and discrimination: an overview. In *Understanding Prejudice and Discrimination*. McGraw-Hill.
Powell, A. (2017) *The Ways of the Soul. A Psychiatrist Reflects: Essays on Life, Death and Beyond*. Muswell Hill Press.

Index

A
abandonment, fear of 16, 88, 197, 216
abortion 79&n
Abrahamic faiths 5, 21, 64, 152, 164
  see also Christianity; Islam; Judaism
acute and transient psychotic disorders (ATPD) 50–51, 200–201, 202
Adam and Eve 13–14, 96–97
adrenaline 16
affect bridge 81
afterlife 32–33&n, 34, 42&n, 67
aggression 16–17, 22, 152, 167, 182–183, 186n, 214&n, 215
alchemy 90–91n, 91
alcohol misuse 75–76, 114, 169
Allport, Gordon 212, 218
aluminium 172
Alzheimer's disease 172
amputee 146, 200
amygdala 16
analytic psychotherapy 30&n
angel, fallen 6
anger 120, 200, 216
animal kingdom 164, 188, 214
anima mundi (world soul) 105
annata ('no-self') 42, 66
Anthony, William 118
antibiotics 127, 157
antidepressants 47, 103, 112, 195
antipsychotics 47, 114
antisepsis 157&n
archetypes 33, 90, 119n
  good and evil 51
  Imago Dei 104n
  Self 60, 119–120, 119n
  soul 106, 205
Arigó, Jose 91–92
Aristotle 204
Aspect, Alain 187–188
Assagioli, Roberto 106
assisted suicide 126
asylums 45–46, 127–128
attention deficit hyperactivity disorder 114, 167
aura (energy field) 31, 91
autistic spectrum disorder 59n, 194
autoimmune disease 214

B
babies 14&n, 15, 26, 58–59, 62, 79–80, 141–143, 145
Baldwin, W.J. 8, 85n
Balint peer groups 137
bardo (spirit realm) 67, 68
Baring, Ann 164, 165
behavioural therapy 47, 48
Bell, John Stewart 187
Bennett, Douglas 127
benzodiazepines 47, 113&n
bereavement 10, 26–27, 30, 33–34, 73, 78–80, 87–88, 107, 206–207

222 INDEX

Bethlem Royal Hospital (Bedlam) 45, 127
Bevan, Aneurin 125
Bible 42
bio-psychosocial model 36
bipolar disorder (manic depressive disorder) 27, 46&n, 114, 157–158, 195
birth 14&n, 26, 28, 96
Blake, William 58
body 73, 74
Boehme, Jakob 43
Bohm, David 95, 96, 163
Bonhoeffer, Dietrich 108
bonobos 213n
boron 172
Brahman 41, 204
brain
    consciousness 44, 112
    enlargement of neocortex 151
    hologram 95–96
    left and right hemispheres 165
    memory 95
    neomammalian 215
    neurophysiology of emotion 16
    paleomammalian 215
    reptilian 215
    triune 215
Buber, Martin 169n
Buddhism 20, 42&n, 59–60n, 61, 65, 66, 67, 94, 141, 152, 182, 183n, 204

C
Campbell, Thomas 204
Care Quality Commission (CQC) 130, 136
care workers 131
case studies *see* clinical examples
categories 212–213
chakras 91&n
chemtrails 172
Chernobyl disaster 173&n, 174
child abuse 168, 171
childhood 96–97, 143, 151, 168
    acquiring self 58–59, 141–143
    attention deficit hyperactivity disorder 114, 167
    ego 215, 216
    family and friends 132–133
    fear of abandonment 16, 216
    first encounters with loss 14–16
    lunar era 177
    mental illness 168, 168–169n
    psychotherapy as adult 75, 77–78, 117
    soul 142–143
    television 167&n
    see also babies; child abuse; parents
Childline 168&n
chimpanzees 213n
Chinese medicine 156
Christianity 21, 42–43, 85, 164–165, 182, 183, 199, 204
    see also God; Jesus Christ
Claridge, Gordon 35–36
classification of mental illness 27, 46&n, 49, 195
clinical examples
    bereavement 33–34, 78–80, 87–88, 206–207
    depression 75, 77, 79, 80, 83, 84
    psychoanalysis 197
    psychodrama 30
    soul-centred psychotherapy 75–88, 75n

soul narratives 206–207
spirit release therapy 1, 35, 85–88
transpersonal therapy 34–35
cognitive–behavioural therapy (CBT) 28, 47
collective unconscious 90
College of Healing 31, 91
community care 116&n, 127&n
compassion 101–102, 107–108
connectedness 134
Conolly, John 45
consciousness 3–4, 8, 10, 97, 104, 151, 162–163, 185, 203
 altered states of 9, 34, 44, 52, 74, 86–87, 106, 199
 brain 44, 112
 collapse of wave function 62, 94–95, 189
 death 32, 65–66
 larger consciousness system 204
 metaphysical view 204
 non-locality 31, 104, 203
 non-ordinary states of (NOSC) 50
 quantum theory 188–189, 203
 soul consciousness 72, 159&n
 transpersonal 90
 universe 94–96, 153
conspiracy theorists 172, 174, 175
Constantine 42
consumerism 17, 18, 52, 158, 169
Copernicus 44, 184
Council of Nicea 42
Creation, story of 214n
Crisp, Arthur 128

Crusades 43, 183
cryptomnesia 67

D
Daoism (Taoism) 21&n, 42, 65, 152, 156
dark matter 163
Davidson, Larry 118
Dawkins, Richard 72&n, 183
death 13, 26–27, 74, 96, 142
 big questions 28
 ego 60, 74
 fear of 60, 74, 82
 hospital errors 127
 life after 32–33&n, 34, 42&n, 67
 soul 74
 substance misuse 169
 as transition 6, 32–34, 78
 see also bereavement; near-death experience; suicide
death instinct 60, 105, 106&n
debts 186&n
defence mechanisms 60, 214–215
deliverance ministry 6–7
delusions 3, 7, 22, 58n
demonic entities 6–7, 85&n
Denning, Steve 134
depression 18, 105, 158, 201–202
 antidepressants 47, 103, 112, 195
 children 168, 168–169n
 clinical examples 75, 77, 79, 80, 83, 84
 electroconvulsive therapy 46–47
 'major depression' in DSM-III 195
 mindfulness 158n
 prevalence 114, 115, 195

recovery 118
self-harm 136–137
soul 190
spirit attachment 4
Descartes, René 44
descriptive psychopathology 195–196
Deus, João de 91–92
diagnosis 25
   diagnostic narrative 194, 195
   mental illness 36, 51–52, 194, 195
   pre-eminence of medical 193–194
direct experience 64–65, 66
disease 27, 194
Dobson, Terry 218–220
doctor–patient relationship 53, 144, 147, 148&n
DSM (*Diagnostic and Statistical Manual of Mental Disorders*) 195
Duncan, Helen 43
Durkheim, Emile 158
dynamic psychopathology 196–198

E

earthbound spirits 2, 5n, 6, 82–84, 86–87
Eastern Orthodox Church 42–43
East, the 20, 41–42
eating disorders 169
Eckhart, Meister 43, 162, 163
ecosystem 152, 157, 170
ego 90, 96, 149, 214, 218
   Buddhism 42
   childhood 215, 216
   death 60, 74
   Maslow's D-needs 135n
   needs wisdom 152
   outward journey of life 142
   past life memory 58, 60&n, 61, 63–64
   possessive pronoun 60n
   science 162, 166, 181
   self-awareness 152
   soul 20&n, 23, 63, 74, 97, 111–112, 120, 148, 175–177, 190, 192
   suffering 19–20, 20&n, 22, 23
Egyptians 41n, 193
Einstein, Albert 2, 162n, 187
elderly people 115&n, 130–131
electroconvulsive therapy (ECT) 46–47
electrons 188
Eliot, T.S. 66, 98
Emerald Tablet 90–91n
Emmott, Stephen 170
emotion, neurophysiology of 16–17
empathy 16, 101, 102, 137, 148, 167
end of life 148–149, 148n
endorphins 16
Englert, François 188
Enlightenment, Age of 44, 164–165
Escher, Maurits, *Drawing Hands* 95&n
ethical issues 7, 36, 47, 116, 197
European Working Time Directive 130, 136
evil 5, 6, 51, 52
extinction, sixth mass 214
extra-terrestrials 64

F

family therapy 28
Field, Nathan 105–106
fight/flight response 15&n, 16, 19, 20, 131

Fitzgerald, Edward 65
fluoxetine (Prozac) 195
foetal distress 14
Fontana, David 94
forgiveness 22–23, 97,
    107–108, 207
Fourier transforms 95
fractals 163
Francis of Assisi 43
Francis Report 127, 130–131
Frankl, Viktor 69n
Freedman, Stuart 187
Freeman, Walter 46n
French wars of
    religion 68&n
Freud, Sigmund 28, 29
    atheist 89–90
    cigar smoking 93
    death instinct 60
    dynamic psychopathology
        196, 197
    group leader 217
    religion 17, 105
    soul 105
    superego 63&n
Fukushima disaster 173–174
functional magnetic resonance
    imaging (fMRI) 2, 101&n

G
Galileo Galilei 44, 184
Gandhi, Mahatma 125n, 186
General Council of Churches,
    5th 42
General Medical Council 132
general practitioner-led
    commissioning groups 132
genocide 22, 199, 213
GeoEngineering Watch 171–172
Gestalt image 174
gnosis 42, 90n
Gnostics 42, 90

God 2, 21, 27, 104&n, 152,
    162, 205
    belief in 17, 40
    Descartes 44
    Godhead 5&n, 65
    Hawking 187
    Imago Dei 90, 104n, 204
    as infinite sphere 141&n
    mystical tradition 43
    Newton 27, 44, 184
    rationalist view 203–204
    solar era 164
    spirituality 26, 73, 189
good, and evil 5, 51, 52
Goswami, Amit 62, 95
Greeks 41&n
greenhouse gases 170&n
Grof, Stanislav 48n, 50
group analysis 29, 74–75, 117,
    134
groups 199, 213, 215, 216–218

H
hallucinations 33–36, 36n,
    200–201, 200n
Hawking, Stephen 166n, 187
healing 40, 89–99
    distant 3, 93–94
    God 27
    hands-on-healing 89n
    medical 93
    medicine 156
    research 91, 92
    spiritual 106
    types of 91–92
    wholeness 26, 31–32, 31n
    wounded psyche 89–99
health, defined 144–145
hearing voices groups 200
heart 75–76, 107, 144, 145–146,
    163, 207&n
    valve 26, 92–93, 155

heaven 5
  and hell 191–192, 191n
Herbert, Ann 190&n
Hermes Trismegistus 90–91n, 141n
hierarchy of needs *see* Maslow
Higgs boson 188
Higgs, Peter 188
High Frequency Active Auroral Research Program (HAARP) 171–173, 172–173n
Hildegard of Bingen 43
Hinduism 20, 41, 59–60n, 141, 182, 183, 187, 204
Hippocrates counsel 156
HIV 157, 158
holographic cosmology 3, 31, 95–96, 104–105, 163
Homo erectus 151
Homo habilis 16, 151, 165–166
Homo neanderthalensis 213
Homo sapiens 14, 16, 63, 64, 74, 151–153, 165, 166, 191, 213–214, 214n, 216
human anatomy 156, 193–194
humanity 151–153, 191
  biological level 151
  civilisation 64
  cultural history 151, 152
  population increase 170–171, 214&n
  psychological level 152
  science and technology 152, 153
  societal level 151–152
  spiritual level 152
  see also Homo sapiens
Huxley, Aldous, *Brave New World* 217n
hypnagogic state 34

I

ICD (*International Classification of Diseases*) 195
  ICD-10 4&n, 9n, 50, 199
Ilibagiza, Immaculee 23
illness 2, 26–27, 32, 96
  denial 144
  recovery 118–119
  self-inflicted 155
  serious 144, 145–146
  short-lived 143
  terminal 148&n
  wholeness and impact of 143–144
  whole patient and doctor 144–146
  see also mental illness
Imago Dei 90, 104n, 204
Improving Access to Psychological Therapies (IAPT) 103n
influenza 157, 158n
informed consent 7
in-patient units 117, 127
Institute of Psychiatry 28
institutions 132–133
insulin coma therapy 46
intellectual empathy 101
internet 167–168, 168n
introjection 78
intuition 96, 162n
intuitives 31, 91
Islam 21, 41, 43, 85, 182, 183&n, 204

J

James, William 35n
Japan
  earthquake 172–173&n
  Fukushima disaster 173–174
Jenner, Edward 157&n
Jesus Christ 3, 42, 182, 188n, 190n, 217–218n

crucifixion 21, 22
kingdom of God 192
love 23, 97
natural world 164
jinn 85
John of the Cross, St. 43, 202
John Radcliffe Hospital 128
Jonestown massacre 199
Joseph, Peter, *Zeitgeist: The Movie* 171
Judaism 21, 41, 43, 182, 204
Judas Iscariot 22
Julian of Norwich 3, 43, 97, 202
Jung, Carl 29, 74–75, 90
    analytical psychology 48
    collective unconscious 90
    death instinct 106&n
    gnostic 90&n
    Imago Dei 90
    Self 60, 119–120
    shadow 21, 216&n
    soul 106, 205, 216n

K
Kabbalah 41
Kafka, Franz 58n
Kaku, Michio 175
Kardec, Allan 5
karma
    collective 22
    law of 20–21, 20n, 42, 64, 74, 93, 94
Karp, Marcia 30
Kastrup, Bernadino 45n
Khayyám, Omar 59, 60, 65, 71, 198
King, Michael 201
King, Truby 15
Koenig, Harold 39, 201
Kraepelin, Emil 27&n, 195
Kundalini experiences 50&n

L
Laing, R.D. 116
liaison psychiatry 28, 194
life 28, 66, 96, 185, 196
    after death 32–33&n, 34, 42&n, 67
    as drama 63
    end of life 148–149
    life force 145
    outward and return journey 142
life instinct 18, 32, 105
light 5, 6, 8, 84
limbic system 16, 19, 215
Lister, Joseph 157&n
lithium 47
lobotomy 46&n
locked-in syndrome 126&n
loss 13, 18, 26–27, 69, 73, 78
love 68, 69&n, 102n, 159, 220
    ego 19–20
    forgiveness 23
    healing power 53
    Maslow's hierarchy of needs 132–133
    mental health professionals 102
    soul love 103–104, 108, 190&n, 218
    unconditional 5, 97, 98, 103, 218
lower astral plane 6
lunar era 164, 165, 177
Luther, Martin 43

M
McGilchrist, Iain 165
MacLean, Paul 215
Maimonides, *Rules of Repentance* 21
Malone, Frank 105–106
mandalas 141

manganese 172
manic depression (bipolar disorder) 27, 46&n, 103, 114, 157–158, 195
Manning, Bradley 175&n
Marx, Karl 17
masculinity 156, 164
Maslow, Abraham, hierarchy of needs 129–138, 130n
   1st level: physiological 130–131
   2nd level: safety and security 131–132
   3rd level: love and belonging 132–133
   4th level: esteem and respect 133–134
   5th level: self-actualisation 135
   being values (B-values) 135
   B-needs 135&n
   caring for carers 135–138
   deficiency needs (D-needs) 135&n
   need for connectedness 134
   NHS 129–138
   transcenders and non-transcenders 135
material realism 2, 9, 44, 63n, 72, 158, 162n, 165–166
Maudsley Hospital 28–29, 117, 126, 127, 128
Medecins Sans Frontières 159
medical model 25, 40, 116, 145
medication 2&n, 27, 40, 47, 113–114, 113n
   see also individual drugs
medicine 2, 25–27
   Chinese 156
   diagnosis 193–196, 202–203
   masculine mind 156
   mederi and *medicina* and healing 156
   soul of 148
   Western 156
meditation 9, 20, 34, 48&n, 52, 74
mediums 3, 4, 5, 9, 43
Mental Health Act 116, 119, 200
mental health, defined 111n
Mental Health Foundation 129
mental health services 127–128, 129, 131, 136–137
mental illness 112–115, 157–158
   children 168, 168–169n
   classification 27, 46&n, 49, 195
   crisis of modernity 49–51
   diagnosis 36, 51–52, 194, 195
   East and West differences 20
   history of care 43, 45–48
   increase in 114–115, 158, 169, 195, 196
   neurochemical model 2
   pharmaceutical narrative 195–196
   physical causation 27, 46, 194
   severe 27, 46, 103, 114, 118, 157–158
   soul 146–147
Merton, Thomas 43
metaphysics 17, 41–42, 203, 204
Milner, Yuri 166n
mind, theory of 59&n
mindfulness-based cognitive therapy 53n, 158&n
ministry of deliverance 85
mirror neurons 101
Mitchell, Edgar 191
monistic idealism 62
monoamine oxidase inhibitors (MAOIs) 47, 113

moral treatment 45
Moreno, Jacob 30&n, 70–71
Moreno, Zerka 146
multidisciplinary teams 116, 128
Muslims 43, 182, 183&n
mystical tradition 43

N
narratives of body, mind and soul 193–209
   authenticity 198–199
   diagnostic narrative 194, 195
   medical diagnosis 193–194, 202
   narratives of science and spirituality meet 203–204
   pharmaceutical narrative 195–196
   power for good or ill 199–200
   psychotic narrative 199
   soul narrative 204–207
   spiritual narrative 200–203, 200n
National Health Service (NHS) 48, 125–139, 158
   caring for carers 135–138
   command and control management 134
   consultants 126, 130, 136
   demoralisation 128–129
   duty of candour 136
   early retirement 131, 137
   efficiency savings 130
   European Working Time Directive 130, 136
   Francis Report 127, 130–131
   gagging clauses 131, 136
   hierarchy of needs 129–138
   history 125–129
   hospital-acquired infections 127
   house officers 130
   managers 129, 131, 133, 138
   medical directors 129
   mental health services 127–128, 129, 131, 136–137
   mistakes 126, 127, 136
   peer group support 136, 137
   porters 133
   scapegoating 132
   staff groups 134
   staff shortages 136, 137
   trusts 128, 129, 131, 136
   ward sisters and consultants 126
   whistle-blowers 131, 136
nation states 217
natural world 163–164, 165, 184
Neanderthals 213&n
near-death experience 3, 6, 52, 65, 74, 94
neocortex 16, 215
Neolithic era 213–214, 216
neti neti ('not this, not that') 65
neurological degenerative disorders 172, 194
neuroscience 2, 112, 113, 156n
neurosyphilis 27, 46
Newtonian physics 9, 27, 44, 45, 91, 94, 153, 161–162, 187
Newton, Isaac 27, 44, 96&n, 175, 184
Nicene Creed 42
Nicholson, David 136
Niebuhr, Reinhold 121&n
nuclear technology 173–174

O
objectivity 3, 44, 45
old age 115&n, 130–131

Orbito, Alex 92
organic conditions 194
Orwell, George 175, 217n
out-of-body states 3, 65, 74, 162

P

paranormal phenomena 32, 52, 90, 91, 162
parents 63
    good parenting 15, 142
    parent/child dynamic in healthcare 198
    parent–infant relationship 101, 132
    therapist in *loco parentis* 30–31
Pargament, Kenneth 202
Pascal, Blaise 43, 96
past life memory 57–72
    acquiring self 58–59, 58n
    crisis of modernity 63–64, 63n
    direct experience 64–65
    examples 67–70, 80–82
    mundane self 61
    past, present and future 59–61, 59–60n
    soul-centred therapy 80–82
    spiritual self 62–63&n
    survival after death 65–67
past life therapy 3, 34, 57, 63, 67, 71, 81–82, 85–88, 106
patients
    importance of religion and spirituality 18, 29, 48, 51–52
    patient journey 117
    whole patient 141–149
Paul the Apostle 201
perinatal trauma 14&n
personality 60, 89, 108
personality disorder 112–113

personhood 117–120, 121
persuasion industry 181–182
pharmaceutical industry 2&n, 40, 195–196
pharmacotherapy *see* medication
phenothiazines 114
photons 187–188
physicalism 162–163, 162n, 203–204
physics
    classical 3–4, 61, 91, 153, 185
    'new' 3
    Newtonian 9, 27, 44, 45, 91, 94, 153, 161–162, 187
    particle 161, 184
Pinel, Phillipe 45
placebo effect 31
Plato 13, 41, 49n, 62n
Poincaré, Henri 96
porphyria 27, 46, 194
possession states 4, 7, 9n, 85, 199
power, abuse of 197
prayer 34, 52, 93–94, 121n
precognition 3
prejudice 211–220, 212n
presence 7, 33, 35&n
presentiment 93–94
Pribram, Karl 95
prodigal son parable 148&n
projection 30&n, 78, 101, 216, 217&n, 218
Proust, Marcel 63
psyche 8, 10, 28, 41n, 60–61
    healing 89–99
    meaning spirit or soul 36, 52
psychiatrists 113
    authority 128
    consultants 116, 128, 130
    conversant with all faith traditions 43
    role of 115–117
    soul narratives 205

spiritual or religious beliefs 18, 40, 52&n, 158
psychiatry 39–55, 119, 143
   20th century 46–49
   diagnosis 194–196
   ethical issues 7, 36, 47, 116, 197
   historical background 40–49
   mental health services 127–128, 129, 131, 136–137
   multidisciplinary teams 116, 128
   paranormal 2–3
   religion 48&n
   research 113
   as science of mind 27–29
   spirituality 25–37, 51–53
psychic surgeons 91–93
psychoanalysis 28, 29, 30, 47–48, 117
   'bottom-up' perspective 62
   dynamic psychopathology 196–197
   ego defences 216
   spirituality 89–90, 105–106
psychodrama 30&n, 70–71, 74–75, 83–84, 117–118, 146
psychodynamic therapy 28, 30–31, 30&n, 78
psychokinesis 3
psychoneuroimmunology 28
psychopathology 3, 200
   descriptive 195–196
   dynamic 196–198
   spiritual pathology 7
psychopaths 15, 101
psychosis 50&n, 127
   acute and transient psychotic disorders (ATPD) 50–51, 200–201, 202
   antipsychotics 47, 114
   psychotic narrative 199
   spiritual crisis 32, 50
   see also bipolar disorder; schizophrenia
psychosomatic medicine 28, 194
psychotherapy 28, 103&n, 105&n, 119, 197–198, 205
   see also individual therapies
Pythagoras 41

Q

quantum mechanics 8, 9
   collapse of wave function 3, 94–95, 188–189
   consciousness 188–189, 203
   entanglement 31, 91
   Jung 90
   non-locality 187–188
   Plato 62n
   reality 3
questions, spiritual 105

R

Rabbeinu Yonah of Gerona, *Gates of Repentance* 21
radical management 134
Randi, James 92
Razzaque, Russell 202
reality
   consensus reality 3, 31–32, 34, 37, 44, 59, 106–107&n
   imagination 2
   material realism 2, 9, 44, 63n, 72, 158, 162n, 165–166
   multiplicity of virtual realities 65, 66
   nature of 2–4
   objectivity 3, 44, 45
   Plato 41

science 184–185
reality testing 106–107&n
recovery 111–123, 202–203
redemption 21, 152
reductionism 156
reincarnation 42, 64, 67
religion 17
    decline in belief 183
    defined 39
    Freud 17, 105
    fundamentalism 217
    intolerance and aggression 182–183
    medicine 27
    mental disorder 201
    psychiatry 48&n
    science 153, 181, 184–186
    soul 182–183
    see also individual religions
Renaissance 44–45
repentance of sins 21
Retreat Hospital, The 45
reverie 34
Rey, Henri 126
Ritalin 167
Rogers, Carl 112, 198
Roman Catholic Church 42–43, 44, 171, 183
Ross, Alistair 105–106
Royal College of Psychiatrists 202
    Spirituality and Psychiatry Special Interest Group (SPSIG) 39, 52–53, 52&n, 158

S
St. Francis' Hospital 127–128
St. George's Hospital 128, 134
samadhi 59–60n
sarcoidosis 81–82
satori 59–60n
Savile, Jimmy 132&n
scapegoating 216
schizophrenia 47, 199
    acute and transient psychotic disorders (ATPD) 50, 51, 201
    causation 114&n, 194
    classification 27, 46&n, 195
    prevalence 114, 157–158
    recovery 118
    spirit release therapy 4, 10
schizotypy 35–36
School of Channelling 91
school phobia 15
schools 15, 132–133
science 17
    'bottom-up' approach 161
    ego 162, 166, 181
    mechanistic science and secularism 184–186
    paradigm shift 8–9, 9n
    religion 153, 181, 184–186
    Renaissance 44–45
    spirit release therapy 2–4
    spirituality 161–165, 187–189, 203–204
    Western 40–41
scientism 181&n, 185n, 213&n
selective serotonin reuptake inhibitors (SSRIs) 47, 113
self 111
    acquiring self 58–59, 59n
    mundane 57, 58, 60, 61
    past life memory 57–72
    self-actualisation 135
    self-awareness 74, 141–143, 151, 152, 188, 203, 215
    spiritual 57, 58, 62–63, 66
Self, Jung on 60, 119–120, 119n
serenity prayer 121n

serotonin and norepinephrine
  reuptake inhibitors
  (SNRIs) 47
shadow 5, 20, 21, 216
shamanic tradition 40, 78
Shipman, Harold 126
Shu, Wun Yi 187
sick role 118
skandhas 66
smallpox 157&n
Snowden, Edward 175&n
sociopaths 173
Socrates 41
solar era 164, 165, 171, 175, 177
somatoform disorders 115
soul
  animal and plant kingdoms
    73–74
  awareness 74, 120, 121,
    189–190, 190n
  body and 141
  conversing with 101–109
  death 74, 97
  defined 5n, 17, 41, 73–74,
    147&n
  ego 20&n, 23, 63, 74, 97,
    111–112, 120, 148,
    175–177, 190, 192
  eye is mirror of 77
  Freud 105
  'going within' 207
  Hinduism 41
  Jung 106, 205, 216n
  loss of 17
  love 103–104, 108,
    190&n, 218
  Maslow's B-needs 135n
  of medicine 148
  modernity 181–192
  Plato 41
  recovery and well-being
    111–123

soul consciousness 72,
  159&n
soul narratives 204–207
soul retrieval 106
suffering 17, 20&n, 21–23,
  22n
Taoism 42
  and technology in 21st
    century 161–179
soul-centred psychotherapy 48,
  73–88, 96, 106, 120
sower, parable of 176&n
space 9, 188
space-time 10, 86–87
Spanish Inquisition 43
speaking in tongues (Toronto
  blessing) 199
spirit, defined 5n, 41, 73
spirit attachment 4, 6–7, 84,
  86–87
spirit presences 91
Spirit Release Forum 1n, 8
spirit release therapy 1–11, 106
  assessment 7&n
  clinical examples 1, 35,
    85–88
  contribution to mental health
    1–11
  demonic possession 85&n
  keeping an open mind 9–10
  science, spirit and nature of
    reality 2–4
  spirit attachment 6–7
  spiritual universe 5
  transformation of 'negative'
    energy 85
spirits
  earthbound 2, 5n, 6, 82–84,
    86–87
  existence of 9
spiritual crisis 18, 32, 49–50,
  51, 202

spiritual emergency 48&n, 50, 52
spiritual healing 106
spiritual history 36–37, 48, 52&n, 202
spirituality 88
　defined 26–27, 39–40, 73, 189
　mental health 48, 201–202
　psychiatry 25–37, 51–53
　psychoanalysis 89–90, 105–106
　science 161–165, 187–189, 203–204
　'spiritual but not religious' demographic 189, 202, 204
　'top-down' approach 162
　in Western history 40–41
Spirituality and Psychiatry Special Interest Group (SPSIG) (Royal College of Psychiatrists) 39, 52–53, 52&n, 158
spiritual life 176&n
spiritual narrative 200–203, 200n
spiritual questions 105
spiritual universe 5, 62
splitting 30&n, 216, 217&n, 218
Stafford Hospital 127, 130–131
stereotyping 213
Stevenson, Ian 67
Stone Mother (hospital) 126–127
Strachey, James 105&n
stress 115, 131
string theory 3
sub-atomic particles 9
subjectivity 2, 44, 45, 59, 62, 203
subject–object divide 90
substance abuse 4, 113, 114, 158, 169
suffering, human 13–24, 29, 69&n

befriending ego 19–20
childhood 14–16
East and West 20–21, 20n, 21n, 42, 152
existential void 18
forgiveness 22–23
individual and collective 21–22
life without soul 17
loss 13, 14, 152
nature of 13–14
neurophysiology of emotion 16–17
pain 13
trauma of birth 14&n
wholeness 147
Sufism 41, 65
suicide 76, 107, 168, 169&n
　assisted 126
　depression 18, 114
　mass 199
　soul narratives 206
　spirit attachment 84
superego 63–64, 63n
Suzuki, Daisetz 199
Swedenborg, Emanuel 5&n, 43
systems theory 28
Szasz, Thomas 196

T

Taiji 42
Talbot, Michael 95–96
tangled hierarchy 95
Taoism *see* Daoism
technology 157, 181–182, 185, 186
　different views 174–175
　left brain 165
　material realism 165–166
　medicine 155, 156
　nuclear technology 173–174

population explosion 170–171, 170n
rise of techno-pathology 166–170, 166n, 167n, 168–169n
science and spirituality 161–165, 162n
and soul in 21st century 161–179
trust breakdown 171–174, 171n, 172–173n
weapons technology 16, 171&n
Teilhard de Chardin, Pierre 43, 204–205, 205n
telepathy 3
therapeuein (therapy) 98
thermodynamics, second law of 187
Tibetan Buddhism 42&n, 67
time 185, 187, 188
space-time 10, 86–87
trance and possession disorders 4, 9n, 52, 85, 199
transference 30&n, 31, 144
transpersonal, defined 104n
transpersonal psychology 48, 104, 105, 120, 162
transpersonal therapy 28, 33–36, 37, 105, 106
tricyclic antidepressants 47, 113
Tuke, William 45
Turoff, Stephen, and Dr Kahn 92–93

U

universe 141
Bohm 95, 163
consciousness 94–96, 153, 163
holographic structure 3, 31, 95–96, 104–105, 163
Newtonian 161–162, 184
spiritual 5, 62
time 185, 187

V

via negativa 65
vibrations 5
video gaming 168
vitamin deficiencies 27, 46

W

wards, locked 127–128
warfare 22, 43, 74n, 159, 164, 171&n, 215n
wave function collapse 3, 32
consciousness 62, 94–95, 189
well-being 111–123, 111n, 135
West, the 17, 20–21, 28, 40–41, 45, 152, 156, 182, 201
wholeness 44, 112, 141–149
discovery of selfhood 141–143
end of life 148–149
healing 26, 31–32, 31n
impact of illness 143–144
mental illness and soul 146–147
patient and doctor 144–146
whole defined 141
Winterbourne View Care Home 131
witchcraft 6, 43
Witchcraft Act 1735 43
Woolger, Roger 67
Wordsworth, William 62, 167
World Health Organization (WHO) 40, 111n, 144–145
World Psychiatric Association, Section on Spirituality and Religion in Psychiatry 40

X
X-rays 91, 161

Y
Yablokov, Alexey 173
yin and *yang* 21, 42

Z
Zen 59–60n, 199, 211

Ingram Content Group UK Ltd.
Milton Keynes UK
UKHW021816270323
419257UK00006B/65